MACRO DIET

Copyright © 2022 by John Wilson
All rights reserved.

No part of this publication may be reproduced, distributed, or transmitted in any form or by any means, including photocopying, recording, or other electronic or mechanical methods, without the prior written permission of the author, except in the case of brief quotations embodied in critical reviews and certain other noncommercial uses permitted by copyright law.

The information contained in this book is not intended and should not in any way replace the doctor-patient relationship or the specialist visit. It is recommended to always seek the advice of your doctor and / or specialists regarding any indication reported. The Publisher does not guarantee or assume responsibility for the information in any form reported.

Author: John Wilson

Independently published

First edition, January 2022

John Wilson

MACRO · DIET ·

COOKBOOK FOR BEGINNERS

The Secrets To Burn Fat By
Eating What You Want Without
Going Hungry

Table of Contents

Introduction	8
Macronutrient Assumptions	8
Different Kinds of Weight Loss	8
The Pitfall of Comparisons	9
It's All About You	11

Chapter 1: Somatotypes

Endomorphs, Ectomorphs, and Mesomorphs	12
Ectomorph	12
Mesomorphs	13
Endomorphs	13
The Challenge of Losing Weight	14

Chapter 2: The Macro Diet

How Does the Macro Diet Work?	15
What Makes the Macro Diet Different?	15

Chapter 3: Benefits of the Macro Diet

The Science Behind the Diet	17
Macronutrients and Energy	17
The Fast Energy System (ATP-PC System)	17
The Medium Energy System (Glycolytic System)	18
The Slow Energy System (Oxidative System)	18
The Benefits of the Macronutrient Diet	19
Psychological Benefits	19
Physical Benefits	19
Lifestyle Benefits	20
How to Indulge and Still See Results	20
How Much Is Too Much?	20

Chapter 4: How to Calculate Macros

The 5 Steps to Macro Success	22
1. Decide Your Goal	22
2. Calculate Your Daily Calories	22
3. Calculate Your Daily Macros	23
4. Plan for Success	25
5. Track Your Daily Numbers	25

Chapter 5: Workout Plan

Weight and Strength Training	26
Exercises	26
Week 1—Day 1	27
How to Do the Exercises	28
1. Air Squats	28
2. Tricep Dips	29
3. Swimmers	30
4. Glute Bridge	31
5. Press Up	32
6. Dead Bug	33
7. Standing Toe Touches	34
8. Cow	35
Week 1—Day 2	36
How to Do the Exercises	37
9. Deadlift	37
10. Bird Dog Plank	38
11. Clams	39
12. Hollow Archs	40
13. Long Lunge	41
14. Calf Raises	42
15. Boat	43
Week 1—Day 3	44
16. Plié Squat	45
17. Split Stance Row	46
18. Donkey Kicks	47
19. Leg Raises	48
20. Single-Leg Box Squat	49
21. Shoulder Press	50
22. Reverse Lunges	51
23. Sphinx	52
Week 2—Day 1	53
How to Do the Exercises	54

24. Single-Leg Raise — 54
25. Lateral Raises — 55
26. Side Lunges — 56
27. Cat-Cow — 57
28. Knee to Elbow Extension — 58
29. Shrugs — 59
30. Wide Squat — 60
31. Cobra — 61

Week 2—Day 2 — 62
How to Do the Exercises — 63
32. Kneeling Shoulder Press — 63
33. Bench Squats — 64
34. Bicycle Crunches — 65
35. High Knees — 66
36. Single Arm Row — 67
37. Leg Abduction — 68
38. Crescent Lunge — 69

Week 2—Day 3 — 70
How to Do the Exercises — 71
39. Plank Hops — 71
40. Front Raises — 72
41. Knee to Chest — 73
42. Flutter Kicks — 74
43. Mountain Climbers — 75
44. Plank Toe Taps — 76
45. Jumping Jacks — 77
46. Baby Cobra — 78

Chapter 6: Foods to Eat and Avoid During Macro Diet

Food Items to Eat on a Macro Diet — 79
Polyunsaturated and Monounsaturated Fats — 79
Food Items to Avoid During a Macro Diet — 80

Chapter 7: Meal Plan

Week 1 — 81
Week 2 — 82
Week 3 — 83

Chapter 9. Breakfast Recipes

1. Blueberry Fat Bombs
2. Cauliflower Poppers
3. Tex-Mex Queso Dip
4. Crispy Parmesan Chips
5. Cheesy Zucchini Triangles with Garlic Mayo Dip
6. Herbed Cheese Chips
7. Bacon & Avocado Omelet
8. Basic Opie Rolls
9. Bacon Hash
10. Bacon & Egg Breakfast Muffins
11. Bacon & Cheese Frittata
12. Baked Apples
13. Parsley Soufflé
14. Tofu Mushrooms
15. Onion Tofu
16. Spinach-Rich Ballet
17. Nut Porridge
18. Pepperoni Egg Omelet
19. Bok Choy Samba
20. Eggs and Ham
21. Bagels with Cheese
22. Breakfast Roll-Ups

Chapter 10. Lunch Recipes

23. Slow Cooked Roasted Pork and Creamy Gravy
24. Grilled Salmon and Zucchini with Mango Sauce
25. Crispy Cuban Pork Roast
26. Garlic Chicken
27. Chicken Broccoli Lunch
28. Keto Barbecued Ribs
29. Chicken Wings and Blue Cheese Dressing
30. Cheesy Chicken Cauliflower
31. Keto Hamburger
32. Turkey and Cream Cheese Sauce
33. Baked Salmon and Pesto
34. Salmon Burgers with Lemon Butter and Mash
35. Chicken Soup
36. Chicken Avocado Salad
37. Turkey Burgers and Tomato Butter
38. Chicken Casserole

39. Keto Chicken with Butter and Lemon
40. Easy Meatballs
41. Buffalo Drumsticks and Chili Aioli
42. Italian Style Eggs
43. Orange and Dates Granola
44. Bacon Muffins
45. Pot Roast with Green Beans
46. Salmon Skewers Wrapped with Prosciutto

Chapter 11. Dinner

47. Baked Zucchini Noodles with Feta
48. Brussels Sprouts with Bacon
49. Bunless Burger—Keto Style
50. Coffee BBQ Pork Belly
51. Salsa Turkey Cutlet and Zucchini Stir-Fry
52. Ranch Turkey with Greek Aioli Sauce
53. Fried Turkey and Pork Meatballs
54. Garlic & Thyme Lamb Chops
55. Whole Chicken with Leek and Mushrooms
56. Mixed Vegetable Patties
57. Keto Meatballs
58. Roasted Leg of Lamb
59. Skillet Fried Cod
60. Steak Pinwheels
61. Salmon Pasta
62. Tangy Shrimp
63. Chicken Thighs with Caesar Salad
64. Grilled Pesto Salmon with Asparagus
65. Jamaican Jerk Pork Roast
66. Slow-Cooked Kalua Pork & Cabbage
67. Chicken Wing and Italian Pepper Soup
68. Pepper, Cheese, Sauerkraut Stuffed Chicken
69. Turkey and Leek Goulash
70. Beef & Broccoli Roast

Chapter 12. Snacks

71. Sweet Onion Dip
72. Keto Trail Mix
73. Eggplant Chips
74. Cold Cuts and Cheese Pinwheels
75. Strawberry Fat Bombs
76. Zucchini Balls with Capers and Bacon
77. Parmesan and Pork Rind Green Beans
78. Kale Chips
79. Roasted Radishes with Brown Butter Sauce
80. Pesto Cauliflower Steaks
81. Crunchy Pork Rind Zucchini Sticks
82. Tomato, Avocado, and Cucumber Salad
83. Avocado Yogurt Dip
84. Keto Bread
85. Creamy Avocado Sauce
86. Loaded Cauliflower Mashed "Potatoes"
87. Healthy Chicken Fritters
88. Cheese Chips and Guacamole
89. Cauliflower "Potato" Salad
90. Perfect Cucumber Salsa
91. Creamy Crab Dip
92. Zucchini Tots
93. Keto Macadamia Hummus
94. Delicious Chicken Alfredo Dip
95. Easy & Perfect Meatballs
96. Cheese Stuffed Mushrooms

Chapter 13. Desserts

97. Chocolate Pudding Delight
98. Raspberry and Coconut
99. Peanut Butter Fudge
100. Cinnamon Streusel Egg Loaf

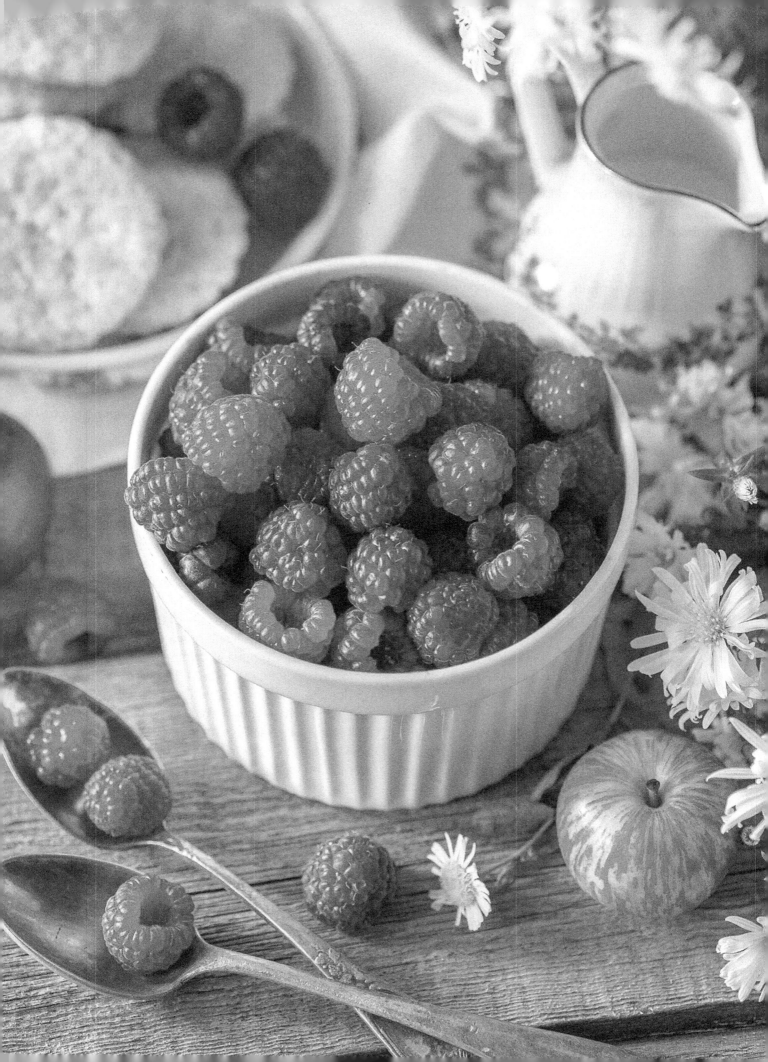

Introduction

When you hear the term "weight loss," what comes to mind? Correct me if I'm wrong, but chances are, you're probably thinking of losing body fat or getting leaner. After all, our clothes don't fit comfortably anymore, because of too much fat in all the "wrong" places.

Adding to that, there are many foolish ways in which people try to lose weight—thinking it's automatically about lowering the numbers on the scale. Some of these include exercising in sauna suits. The quickest way to lose weight is by dehydrating one's body, but it's an unhealthy way of doing it. Given that it's very easy to lose weight through dehydration, the flip side is true: It's very easy to gain it back!

The principle behind this is to make a person sweat excessively and, in the process, lose weight quickly. An even more reckless idea is not drinking water while preventing the supposedly lost weight from coming back.

This represents an unhealthy way of trying to lose weight regardless of the somatotype. Dehydration is one of the worst things that can happen to a person's body—even while at rest.

The worst that can also happen with persistently exercising in a dehydrated state is organ failure. When that happens, it's game over.

Extreme crash diets severely restrict caloric intake to lose the most weight in the shortest time possible. And while some diets don't do this, they can still be considered crash diets because they severely limit or eliminate specific types of macronutrients or food groups (the most popular is restricting carbs). They are impractical and go against the human body's natural mechanisms, requiring too much of a person's limited willpower reserves. And just like meteors entering the Earth's atmosphere, most people who go through crash diets eventually crash and burn. In the end, they don't just burn out but regain the weight that they lost—and even more.

I'm not saying that crash diets fail "all the time." However, a person's chances of successfully and healthily losing weight and keeping it off are very slim because of the reasons stated earlier.

Macronutrient Assumptions

We will talk about macronutrients in more detail later. For now, know that they refer to the three main kinds of calories: Carbohydrates, protein, and dietary fats.

By macronutrient assumptions, we mean applying the same ratios to everybody with the same weight goals. As you will learn later, this is one key to successfully losing weight, and keeping it off.

Different Kinds of Weight Loss

You can still go down several notches in clothing sizes without losing weight, or you may even gain a few pounds. How's that possible?

Again, let's go back to the fundamental goal of losing weight, which is body fat loss. If your clothes no longer fit you, the chances are high that it's because of accumulated body fat. However, if you lose body fat and build muscle along the way, it's possible to fit into your old clothes while maintaining your body weight or even slightly increasing it.

Body fat tissue has a density of 0.03 oz. per 0.03 fl oz., while muscle tissue has a density of 0.04 oz. per 0.03 fl oz. To put it in layman's terms, if you lose 41 oz. of body fat but gain 31 fl oz. of muscle tissue during the same period, you may still weigh the same. However, your waistline and general body size will shrink. It's because, in terms of volume, it takes less muscle volume to achieve the same weight compared to body fat. You may still weigh the same in this example, but in terms of tissue volume, you would have lost more fat tissue (41 fl oz.) than you've gained in muscle mass (31 fl oz.). Now, can you see the importance of ensuring that you lose mostly body fat instead of water and muscle mass?

Another reason as to why you can weigh the same but look leaner is because of the way muscles and body fat determine how your body looks. If you gain 10 pounds of body fat, you'll look bigger, softer, and more out of shape. Contrast that to gaining 10 pounds of muscle mass. Doing so makes you look much fitter, leaner, and toned.

Another reason to ensure that you lose mostly body fat and minimal muscle mass is your metabolism. Between the two, muscles are the more metabolically active cells in your body. Having more muscle mass can increase your resting metabolic rate, which means that you can burn more calories (and, consequently, body fat) even while physically resting. If you lose more muscle mass than body fat, your metabolism will slow down and make it even more difficult to burn calories and lose weight.

Also, having excess body fat levels significantly increases your health risks. Obesity puts you at risk for life-threatening conditions, such as heart attack, hypertension, liver cirrhosis, and diabetes, to name a few. It also increases your chances of physical injuries because the excess weight puts too much chronic strain on your joints and muscles.

You see, losing weight can be a worthy goal, but it shouldn't be your primary goal. The most important benefit of losing excess weight is optimal health and wellness. What's the point of looking fit if you're unhealthy?

When relating to a person's overall condition, we use the terms health and fitness. We can be healthy but not fit or be fit and unhealthy.

Now, I hope that your paradigm about losing excess weight has changed. If done right, losing weight can lead to automatic improvements in health. You will learn how to lose weight healthily and sustainably. You won't just look much better, but you'll also be much healthier.

The Pitfall of Comparisons

Comparing your body weight and measurements while trying to shed off excess body fat can be a double-edged sword. That is why it's also essential to learn the proper way to compare your progress.

Why should you compare? Unless you do this correctly, you won't be able to track or monitor your weight loss progress properly. Comparison entails evaluating your weight and measurements using two specific benchmarks. The benchmark you use for comparison will determine whether you're comparing your numbers correctly or incorrectly.

You must compare your current numbers to your previous ones. Put simply, compare your current body weight to how much you weighed the week before. By doing so, you'll know whether you have lost or gained weight during the week.

Now, there's an incorrect way to compare your weight, and you must know this to avoid comparison pitfalls and maximize your chances of successfully shedding excess fat.

Never compare your body weight and measurements with those of others! That is a definite recipe for discouragement, false hope, and failure. Why is that?

Your body composition, genetics, personal circumstances, and history differ from mine and everybody else's. All these factors (and more) have a say when it comes to how fast or slow you'll be able to lose body fat and the strategies and tactics required to keep them off. So, comparing your weight loss development to professional fitness competitors is neither realistic nor practical.

For one, fitness competitors make a living from their physical fitness and conditioning. Their day job entails exercising and following strict diets all day, every day. These aren't side projects or hobbies—these are their "livelihoods." As such, they can dedicate all their time and resources to exercising and dieting in ways that most people may find extreme or impractical.

As a result, they can achieve such high physical fitness levels and low body fat much faster. Also, it's much easier for them to maintain how they look. If you are not a professional fitness competitor, it will take you more time to lose excess body fat. If you compare your progress with such people, you will never measure up. It's a guaranteed recipe for discouragement and, eventually, quitting.

Another thing to consider when making the proper comparisons is circumstances. Weigh yourself and take body measurements at the same set time of the day and under the same set of circumstances.

For example, you may choose to measure yourself first thing in the morning every Monday before eating or drinking anything and after you have been to the bathroom. When you weigh yourself in this way, the number you will get may be considered your "clean body weight"; for example, weight in food and drinks will not be counted.

But if you weigh yourself every week at different times of the day, you won't be able to compare apples to apples. Now, suppose you weighed 190 pounds last Monday morning (after going to the bathroom but before eating and drinking anything), and then weighed 193 pounds this Monday evening. You'd think that you had gained more pounds over the week, despite dieting and exercising. If you believe this, you may adjust your diet and exercise to burn more body fat in ways that may become unproductive—or unhealthy.

For example, you may severely cut your calories even further and exercise longer, harder, and more frequently for the rest of the week—overdoing things and severely affecting your long-term weight loss success.

In this example, your body weight last Monday morning is considered your clean body weight. Most pounds/ounces represent your absolute weight, i.e., the weight of food and drinks were not counted.

But, your body weight this Monday evening includes the food and drinks you've consumed throughout the day, less the ones you've excreted already. That means part of your body weight isn't yours, but comes from the things you've consumed throughout the day.

You can't say you've gained weight when there's a high possibility that the additional pounds were not absolute body weight. Therefore, it's important to weigh yourself at the same time of the day and under the same set of circumstances.

More than just weighing yourself, you must also measure your body fat levels because the goal here is to shed excess body fat and not just body weight for the sake of weighing less. Remember, if you lose more body fat than muscle in terms of volume, you may still look thinner or leaner while gaining a pound or two. This is possible because muscles have a higher density than body fat does; therefore, gaining more muscle can help you look fitter and leaner.

By taking both body weight and body fat level measurements, you can determine if you're losing the right weight, i.e., body fat. If you lost three pounds last week, but your body fat levels went up from 23% to 25%, that's not a good indicator. It means the weight you lost is either water weight or, worse, muscle mass. Suppose it "is" muscle mass, and the trend continues. Thus, your metabolism will eventually slow down, and the chances of you losing more weight and keeping it off decreases.

The most accurate way of measuring body fat levels involves using highly specialized scanning equipment that may cost you at least $100 a pop. If you plan to monitor your body fat levels weekly, you may lose more than just body weight; your bank account may also get leaner!

The cheapest way to measure body fat is by using body fat calipers. Before the invention of sophisticated body fat measuring equipment, this was the gold standard. It was the only standard. The challenge of this relatively cheap and easy method is the difficulty of its use. It requires pinching different areas of your body—several of which are pretty tricky to do yourself—and measuring the thickness of the skin folds. Electronic body fat measuring equipment proved to be much more accurate.

So, the choice appears to be either breaking the bank or settling for a cheap (but difficult to use) method to measure body fat. Fortunately, there's another option. Today, it's easy to buy affordable and relatively accurate equipment that uses electrical impedance to do the job. These include digital weighing scales with body fat analyzers or handheld electronic devices that do the same thing.

Whether using a digital body fat analyzer, calipers, or a costly testing service, 'consistency' matters most. Like the need to weigh yourself at the same time of day and under the same conditions, the accuracy of your progress tracking requires you to use the same piece of body fat level measuring equipment each time. You must track the increases or decreases in your body fat level consistently. If you use a caliper to measure body fat levels this week, then use a digital weighing scale that uses electrical impedance next week; it's pretty much like measuring your waistline using the metric system today and inches later.

Body fat numbers that decrease and increase because you're using different measuring devices are neither accurate nor comparable. If you use a digital weighing scale or a handheld body fat analyzer, you must be consistent in terms of the time of day and circumstances under which you use it. This is because your body's hydration levels can significantly influence the readings you'll get from this equipment. For the most accurate readings possible, measure your body fat level first thing in the morning, after you go to the bathroom, and before drinking or eating. That way, the readings that you'll get will be comparable and consistent.

It's All About You

Before we proceed any further in your Macro Diet journey, always keep in mind that it's all about you. Compare your results, or lack thereof, only to your last numbers and not anybody else's. You are not other people, and other people are not you, so don't expect yourself to progress at the same pace as others. Keep your eye on the prize and, more importantly, on your weight and fat loss developments.

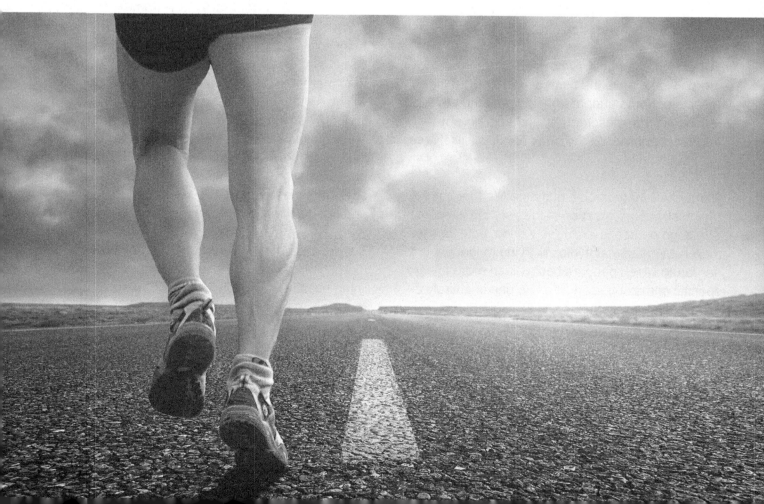

Chapter 1: Somatotypes

While this is a book about losing weight healthily and effectively, what sets it apart from other books is emphasizing on somatotypes. Are you an endomorph, or is your somatotype something else? Whether or not you already have an idea, let's look at somatotypes.

Endomorphs, Ectomorphs, and Mesomorphs

"Somatotype" refers to a person's physique type and body shape. This term is used as a specific system of classifying people's physical shapes developed by an American psychologist named William Sheldon. According to the system, there are three extreme body types under which people can be classified: "Endomorphic," "mesomorphic," and "ectomorphic."

A person's somatotype is typically expressed as a three-digit number. The first digit refers to a person's endomorphy, the second digit relates to their mesomorphy, and the last number is related to ectomorphy. Each number lies between one and seven, with one being the lowest and seven the highest.

For example, a person who is an extreme endomorph would have the number 711. The 1st digit reflects extreme endomorphy (7), and the other two reflect minimal mesomorphy and ectomorphy. An extreme ectomorph, on the other hand, will likely reflect the number 117.

Remember that extreme numbers like these are practically nonexistent or, at the very least, scarce. In effect, no person is exclusively endo, ecto, or mesomorph. What somatotyping is trying to identify is the degree to which people's bodies lean more toward specific somatotypes. Just as no one is entirely extroverted or introverted, specific somatotypes are not more dominant for any one person.

But more than just the general shape of the body, your somatotype also describes your physical, genetic predisposition, among which is your body fat levels. For this reason, you'll need to diet and train in specific ways that are compatible with maximizing your ability to shed body fat and keep it off in the long run. So, let's look at each somatotype in more detail.

Ectomorph

People with this somatotype are generally blessed with a fast metabolism. Their bodies can burn more calories even while at rest compared to meso and endomorphs. They also have a slight build.

Because of their generally smaller size and faster than average metabolism, ectomorphs find it hard to gain weight regardless of body fat or muscle mass. If you have a friend or family member who eats like a horse but is as slim or lean as a pole, you're looking at an ectomorph. An excellent example of ectomorphs is marathon runners, i.e., slight builds, relatively ripped bodies, and minimal muscle mass. Ectomorphs also tend to have narrow shoulder blades and flat chests. They're also naturally lean.

Because of their generally small frames, relatively lightweight, and low body fat percentage compared to muscle mass, ectomorphs tend to be ideal in speed and endurance sports. Again, look no further than marathon runners and track and field athletes. It will be hard to sprint fast if you're not optimally lean. To jump as high or as long as possible, which is the case in events like the high jump, pole vault, and long jump, you must be the lightest possible version of yourself. A 10-pound increase in body weight can spell the difference between winning the gold medal and not qualifying at all.

But because of their relatively light weight, ectomorphs aren't ideal athletes for combat and weightlifting events. This is because their relatively fast metabolism means that they have less than average muscle mass, which is very important for these sports. Ectomorphs need to focus more on heavy weightlifting and minimize (or even ditch) cardio exercises to build muscle mass.

On the nutritional side, ectomorphs also need to eat a lot more than mesomorphs and endomorphs to gain weight. And if the emphasis is on gaining muscle mass, they must eat even more. This is mainly because weightlifting burns more calories than cardio workouts.

One advantage of this somatotype is eating anything without regard for gaining weight easily. Ectomorphs can tolerate high carbohydrate diets with their speedy metabolism, which maximizes physical performance, and is especially useful when lifting weights.

For ectomorphs who are dead serious about gaining weight, their best bet would be foods with very high caloric densities. Supplements and meal replacement products that pack a lot of caloric wallop in significantly smaller servings can be an ectomorph's best friend. These include high-calorie protein shakes and the like.

Mesomorphs

A person with this type of body is one who typically has a medium-built frame and bone structure. They also tend to have considerable levels of lean body mass and, as a result, are more naturally athletic than most people. Typically, mesomorphs gain muscle mass much more easily because of their body's natural ability to produce lots of growth hormones. Because muscles are much more metabolically active than other types of cells in the body, mesomorphs are naturally lean and muscular, unlike ecto and endomorphs.

It's easy for them to bulk up with weight or resistance training, given their genetic predisposition to building muscle. They quickly see results, and as such, have a genetic advantage over endo and ectomorphs.

Along with quick muscle gains comes increased body fat. That's why mesomorphs need to eat the right macronutrient proportions to complement their training.

Nutritionally speaking, mesomorphs can moderately tolerate carbohydrates. This means they may eat relatively more carbohydrates but only within the context of physical training and post-training recovery. Otherwise, they must moderate the number of carbohydrate calories they consume to avoid gaining more body fat than muscle.

Endomorphs

The typical endomorph body is genetically predisposed to having higher body fat levels and tends to have a softer body mass. This is because among the three somatotypes, being an endomorph means having a significantly slower metabolism than ecto and mesomorphs. One of the main reasons for this is they're more insulin dominant—a key factor in quickly gaining body fat and having difficulty losing it.

Fortunately, along with ease of gaining body fat comes a relatively easier time gaining muscle mass. But unlike mesomorphs, endomorphs need to eat and train in specific ways to maximize muscle mass gains and minimize body fat accumulation. That's why being an endomorph with excess weight isn't necessarily a lifelong prison sentence.

Speaking of physical traits, the most common ones associated with being an endomorph include:

• Minimum muscle definition, if any, and a generally soft body

• A naturally round-shaped body

• A propensity to gain body fat easily

• A large bone structure

• Slow metabolism

Despite being more challenged in achieving and maintaining relatively healthy body weight and lean body, endomorphs can still successfully achieve these goals. With the correct nutritional approach and training strategy, fat loss and maintaining a relatively lean body is not an impossible dream.

The Challenge of Losing Weight

You've probably tried your best to lose excess weight using a variety of diets and exercise programs. And still, you haven't lost those pounds and inches. Why?

Mainly because your genetic disposition is to be insulin dominant instead of being growth hormone dominant, it's essential to understand the role of insulin and growth hormones play in your metabolism to understand its repercussions on your weight loss efforts.

Insulin is a hormone produced by your pancreas, and it primarily regulates blood sugar levels. When you eat, your body digests and breaks this food down into glucose—the primary fuel your body uses for daily activities. After successfully doing so, glucose enters your bloodstream to be distributed among your body's cells to provide the necessary nutrients and energy for survival.

Depending on the amount of glucose that enters your bloodstream at any given time, your blood sugar level will rise. If too much glucose enters it too fast, your blood sugar level spikes or increases significantly and quickly. When this happens, your pancreas secretes insulin to bring your blood sugar level down quickly.

At first glance, this seems to have nothing to do with weight loss or weight gain. But when insulin acts on excess blood sugar to normalize its level, it converts it into glycogen for storage in the liver. The organ's capacity for glycogen storage is limited. The glucose overspill is then converted into body fat.

This isn't the only bad news. When blood sugar spikes and crashes become the norm rather than the exception, your pancreas goes under increasing stress to produce more insulin. At one point, your body may develop what is called insulin resistance. Under this condition, the amount of insulin needed to bring blood sugar down to normal levels increases because the body starts to develop "resistance towards it."

If left uncontrolled, it will eventually result in non-responsiveness to insulin, chronically high blood sugar levels, and eventually diabetes.

More than just significantly impacting your body fat levels, being insulin dominant can also lead to a higher risk of diabetes. That's why part of the Macro Diet's nutritional strategy is to eat the right amount of macronutrients, especially carbohydrates.

The other reason why losing weight can be more challenging is the naturally slower metabolism, whether the individual has a sweet tooth or not. Metabolism refers to the rate at which the body can burn calories from the food and drinks consumed daily.

The faster one's metabolism is, the greater the required daily calories are. But a slower metabolism means fewer daily required calories. This means that a person with a fast metabolism will not gain weight even after eating a tub of ice cream in one sitting. On the other hand, even just a cone of ice cream can lead to weight gain for a person with a slow metabolism.

Another reason why many people appear to fail in their weight loss goals is because of discouragement or even a simple lack of motivation. Because many of them use inappropriate or ineffective weight loss strategies for their somatotype, they may have gained significant weight over the years. Being heavyset or overweight can make regular exercise more challenging for them. They'll need to use a lot more willpower just to start a diet and a fitness program. Because they experience little to no results compared to the two other somatotypes in the same timeframe, their willpower reserves eventually dry up, and they become demotivated. Thus, they inevitably fail to lose excess weight.

Now, these three challenges appear to make successful weight loss and maintenance impossible. Still, with the proper nutritional and training strategies, you'll be able to accomplish your body weight and fitness goals and keep the fat you lost from creeping back.

Chapter 2: The Macro Diet

Diets are named for many things, such as the person who created them or even when the diet supposedly originated. The macro diet could have fallen under either of these. Still, the diet's name has persisted throughout millennia, and its historical effectiveness speaks for itself.

How Does the Macro Diet Work?

The macro diet focuses on balance, as mentioned above. The diet is meant to focus on four main food groups (carbohydrates, vegetables, proteins, and fats) to create an optimally healthy person. The diet believes in balancing your body and physical activity to make you the healthiest possible individual. Your body is a living and working machine that needs maintenance and fuel to operate at peak capacity. The macro diet focuses on the fuel aspect to feed the body the nutrients it needs appropriately.

That's not to say the diet lacks flavor. Macro diet foods can be some of the best tasting foods available. The options and the varieties are limitless for those who want to follow this diet. The fact that each meal is balanced for health also means that it's balanced for flavor. Imagine being excited to eat every meal because of how delicious it will be as well as good for you. That's how you'll stick to this diet and do so without any complaints. There are other reasons, too, considering the differences between the macro diet and other diets.

What Makes the Macro Diet Different?

The goal of the diet is to achieve balance in your diet by focusing on the most critical aspects of the food we eat every day. The macro diet is also standard in many countries around the world where people are leading happy and healthy lives simply by following the eating traditions of their country. That's not to say you can't benefit from this diet if you don't live in those parts of the world. All you need to do is change how you shop and view food in your area. So long as you have access to a supermarket or can reliably attain your everyday products, a basic kitchen setup, and the desire to see results, you can begin and will benefit from the macro diet.

The other thing that makes this diet different from the others is that it's not a fad. This is a scientifically proven diet that continues to help people all over the world. It's the only one with consistent results with no negative repercussions for those who decide to pursue it for the sake of their health. Make no mistake: The macro diet isn't meant to be a trend. This isn't something you can do for a few months and then tell your friends not to do it after you've abandoned it because you felt it wasn't for you.

The macro diet is accessible for just about anyone on any budget. It is for everyone because there are no restrictions except for those you put on yourself for personal or health reasons. Even in those cases, the macro diet can be followed because it is so versatile. Even if you're a hardcore vegan, the diet can be filled with vegan and vegetarian recipes. Even if a recipe calls for an animal product, you should know how to substitute them to create your own version of the dish.

Forget about calorie counting as you know it, too. Every person has different caloric intake needs. It's more important to balance what you're eating rather than count how many calories each meal contains. Caloric values are always mentioned in the recipes, as well as portion sizes. Still, these aren't there to measure how many calories you eat. They are there for nutritionists and other health professionals to understand which recipes would work better for their patients on a given day. Generally, it's always best to consult your doctor before starting any diet or exercise regimen so you can identify your needs. The calories are there to help you with those needs rather than restrict your choice of what to eat.

That said, without knowing your physical activity, age, gender, exercise habits, muscle mass, body mass index, supplements taken, genetic factors, weather, and pregnancy status, it's impossible to know the specifics that your body needs without consulting your doctor. That doesn't mean that you can't start the macro diet without this information. It just means the ideal way of following the diet for your needs is unknown until you speak to your doctor. Suppose you know your own conditions and limitations. In that case, you can use the formula in the next section to determine your caloric needs. It's important to reiterate that nothing will replace a medical professional's guidance, so take the following section as more of a guide than a hard rule.

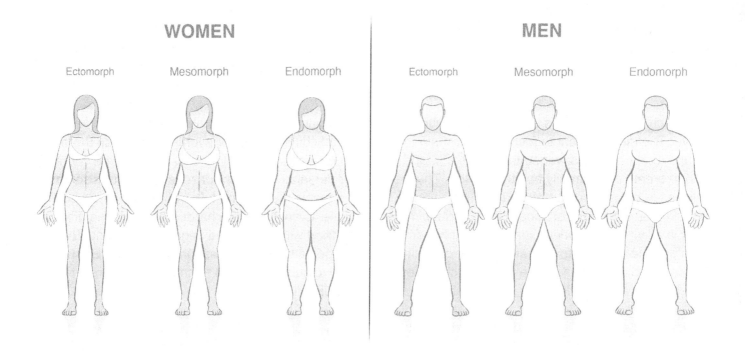

Chapter 3: Benefits of the Macro Diet

There are many different diet plans available, and with so many to choose from, it's important to choose the one that's a good fit for your individual lifestyle and preferences. The macronutrient diet is easily adaptable to any dietary schedule, lifestyle, and preference. This chapter will take you through both the science of the macronutrient diet and also the wide range of benefits that this flexible diet offers. You'll also learn about your body's different energy-burning cycles and how properly integrating your macronutrients throughout the day can help your progress.

The Science Behind the Diet

The macronutrient diet doesn't always make sense. After all, you've probably been told your entire life that you can only lose weight by eating "clean" foods. Candy bars and pizza? Those foods make you fat. If you want to lose weight, you can only eat grilled chicken, sweet potatoes, egg whites, spinach, and asparagus.

This information is well-meaning—most of the time. A lot of so-called experts truly believe that you must eat these clean food sources if you want to lose weight and get healthy. This book isn't trying to show that eating indulgent foods is bad, not by any means. A diet full of whole foods will have significantly more nutritional benefits than a regimen full of processed and packaged foods.

The macronutrient diet does not "require" you to eat junk food regularly; it simply allows it. The macro diet, or flexible diet, refers to tracking your food, being precise with your macronutrient intake, and giving yourself the freedom to choose what foods to eat. Flexible dieting could be applied to carb cycling, a clean eating regimen, the Paleo diet, a ketogenic diet, or any other diet really.

You must understand that the "clean eating" diet isn't the "only way." It's very possible, and in fact more sustainable in the long term, to eat the foods you enjoy in moderation regularly. The idea of giving up any one food forever is scary, but if you know you can enjoy your favorite foods whenever you want, guilt-free, so long as you account for them, it makes the prospect of long-term dieting much easier.

Macronutrients and Energy

A calorie is simply a measure of energy, excess calories are stored as body fat, and calories come from protein, carbohydrates, and fat. That's a good basic understanding, but it's time to get a little more in-depth with that and look at the various ways your body uses energy and which macronutrients support those energy systems. The idea that excess calories will be stored for later usage is the big picture; now, it's time to look at the details.

There are three categories of energy systems in your body—complex processes that produce the required energy for whatever activity you're doing. Within these categories are various subcategories, but unless you're concerned with elite levels of human performance optimization, the subcategories aren't particularly important to understand. For fat loss and nutrition, you just need to know the basics of the big three systems.

It's very important to look at exercise as a means of improving your body's health—because it is. If you see it as punishment or strictly as a way to burn calories, it will be much harder to enjoy it and make it a sustainable habit. Remember, you are getting stronger and setting yourself up to live a longer, healthier life. Burning extra calories is just a nice side effect.

Whether you're sleeping in bed or sprinting up a hill, one of the three energy systems is at work. The scientific names for these systems are the ATP-PC system, glycolytic system, and oxidative system, but just think of them as the fast, medium, and slow energy systems.

The Fast Energy System (ATP-PC System)

This fast energy system is your maximum effort, short-duration system. It can supply an intense burst of energy for around 10–12 seconds before it runs out of steam and the next system takes over. This is used when you are jumping, lifting something very heavy, or doing a fast and short run, like sprinting across a basketball court.

In terms of nutrition, you don't really need to worry about this one too much. Just know it exists. Because it's such a short burst of energy, it uses something called "adenosine triphosphate" (ATP), which is made and stored in your muscle cells. As long as you're getting enough calories and nutrients, you'll have plenty of ATP available.

The Medium Energy System (Glycolytic System)

Next up is the glycolytic system, or medium energy system, which is pretty complicated. All you need to know is that this system powers your moderate-to-high intensity, short-duration activities, such as sprinting, lifting weights, playing a sport, or anything else that would feel like a workout. The medium energy system kicks in after about 10 seconds, when the fast energy system runs out and works for slightly longer—although it still runs out fairly quickly.

This energy system primarily uses glucose produced from stored glycogen. To put it in simpler terms, glucose is a simple sugar molecule, so this system is running on sugar. When you consume carbohydrates, they are stored as glycogen in your muscles. Glycogen is readily available for your body to use during exercise, and while the body can produce it naturally using protein or fat, nothing is faster.

Those carbohydrates, in the form of glycogen, are later broken down further into simple sugar molecules that fuel the glycolytic (or medium) energy system. This is why athletes talk about carb-loading before a race or a big sporting event; they want to make sure their glycogen stores are filled, so their bodies have plenty to draw from.

Even if you aren't an athlete, consuming carbohydrates around your workout is important for maximum performance. Now that you understand how this system works, you should be able to see why. Giving your body readily available fuel in the form of glycogen is essential if you want to run at your highest level.

So what happens if there is no glycogen in the muscles to be used? If you remember, you learned that carbohydrates are not essential for life. If they aren't essential, and you aren't consuming any and storing them as glycogen, how does this medium energy system operate? Well, your body can undergo the complex process of gluconeogenesis. This process involves breaking down stored muscle tissue, ripping it apart, and converting it to glucose. This is a much slower way to get glucose and is not optimal.

If you regularly exercise intensely, your best bet is to include carbs in your diet, at least on workout days. You "can" work out without carbs, but your performance will suffer, as you won't have that glycogen ready for easy access. Think of your glycogen stores as a fuel tank for the car that is your body and carbohydrates as the fuel. Without fueling up, you'll have a difficult time operating at peak efficiency for any length of time.

The Slow Energy System (Oxidative System)

The last of the big three you need to know about is the oxidative system. This is the slow energy system, and it provides a sustained release of energy for low-to-moderate activities that last a bit longer. Long runs, swimming, hiking, hot yoga, yard work—these are all activities that are more intense than your resting state but can be sustained for a long time.

This system uses a mixture of carbohydrates and fats for fuel. While carbohydrates are still important and will benefit your body when it's using the oxidative system, they aren't quite as important as they are to the medium energy system.

If you regularly go on long walks, hikes, or swim laps for your exercise, carbs are optional for you. They may help, but your body can also run just fine off of fat during these long-duration exercises. The choice is yours. Carbs are very useful during moderate-to-high intensity, short-duration exercises, but with these easier forms of exercise, carbs aren't quite as important.

The Benefits of the Macronutrient Diet

A flexible diet is adaptable to any lifestyle and schedule. Where most diets are focused solely on fat loss, the macronutrient diet works with any goal, whether that goal is fat loss, muscle gain, athletic performance, or simply general health.

The next section will provide real-life examples of how this diet can be the perfect fit for any lifestyle. It may sound too good to be true; after all, diets aren't supposed to be fun, right?

Well, not only can this diet be fun, but it's also the best option for a sustainable, healthy plan that you could realistically follow for the rest of your life. Most diets are too restrictive and aren't meant to last longer than twelve weeks. If you put in the time to understand and learn how flexible dieting works, you'll know how to eat for optimal health for the rest of your life.

Psychological Benefits

The number one benefit of this diet and the reason so many people find it sustainable for the long haul is the lack of restriction. It's not a free-for-all diet, and you do need to exercise some self-control and portion control, but you can still eat any food you want, so long as it fits your macro targets for the day.

Freedom to choose what foods you want to eat is a refreshing approach to dieting and the one that will be the most sustainable. Basic psychology reveals that humans tend to be more drawn to what they aren't supposed to have. If someone walked up and told you that you could never eat your favorite food again, how much more would you crave it? Even if you didn't want it that badly before, knowing it would be off the table forever probably makes you want it.

With flexible dieting, this is never an issue. You don't have to have one last cheat day before giving up bread for the summer. You don't have to skip dessert at social events. With the macronutrient diet, if you plan ahead of time and make the correct adjustments, any food you can imagine can fit your plan.

Once you get this diet down, which does take practice and a bit of mental training, if you've dieted before, you can start to remove the guilt you may associate with eating "junk" food. It's very common to see someone on a diet slip up and eat something they weren't supposed to, feel guilty and ashamed, and then just blow off the diet completely, promising to start again on Monday. This is a bad cycle and an unnecessary negative association with food. Flexible dieting allows you to break this cycle for good if you take the time to practice it and make it work.

Physical Benefits

From a physical health perspective, flexible dieting is a great way to get in shape and ensure you're getting the proper nutrients you need without any guesswork. The precision required means that if you set up your numbers and food sources properly, you can give your body exactly what it needs to feel and look good day after day.

Other diets tend to take a broad approach; they ask you to eliminate certain food groups, try to control your portions, and hope for the best. Sometimes this works, and sometimes it doesn't, but they don't always ensure you're actually getting the right nutrients.

Simply telling you to cut out processed foods, for example, doesn't mean you'll understand the ins and outs of nutrition and make sure you're eating the right foods every day. Because flexible dieting requires you to get involved and pay attention to what's in all the foods you're eating, you'll learn a lot about nutrition and what's actually in various foods as you begin tracking.

As far as body composition is concerned, flexible dieting is the most precise way to control your food intake and make small adjustments as needed. If you always have an idea of exactly where your calories are at, as well as your individual macronutrients, it's easy to make a small adjustment, like removing 30 grams of carbs from your daily intake, adding 10 grams of fat, or things like that. An untracked diet makes it impossible to be precise, and this precision is needed to push through plateaus and continue to see results.

Lifestyle Benefits

The number one benefit of the flexible diet is that as long as you track your macros, you can eat any foods you want at any time of the day, and if the numbers add up, you'll still see the changes in your body that you desire. No other diet out there allows this sort of customization to your individual lifestyle.

Time is the biggest reason given for why people can't get in shape. Exercising takes time, cooking healthy meals takes time, and most people have very full schedules. Between work, a social life, and family time, the idea of cooking three to four healthy meals every day and finding time to exercise throughout the week can seem nearly impossible.

With flexible dieting, you can build a meal plan that fits your schedule. If you find that you have a very busy morning with no time to eat, you can grab a light snack and save most of your calories for later in the day. If you wake up starving, you can eat a huge breakfast. If you work split shifts or are a student with an irregular schedule, you can simply eat whenever you have a minute to sit down and make the numbers work.

There is no rigid schedule or strict meal plan to follow. Every part of the macronutrient diet can be tailored to your exact needs and preferences.

How to Indulge and Still See Results

On to the most fun part of the book: How to eat all the foods you love without sabotaging your progress. This may be the only diet in existence that not only allows you to eat your favorite foods, but encourages them. You also shouldn't have to use negative words like "cheat meals"; these meals and snacks should fit into your diet without causing you to miss your macros, and as such, are perfectly acceptable.

The biggest problem people have is regarding health concerns. You'll hear lots of false claims about artificial sweeteners, processed foods, GMOs, and other "evils" of the food industry. It may be worth addressing those things if you're in the medical field or you have a special condition, but those are irrelevant for most people. Are artificial sweeteners healthy? Probably not. However, their dangers are severely overstated, and unless you're consuming ten cans of diet soda a day, you should be fine. The other fact people tend to overlook is that carrying excess body fat is far unhealthier than whatever trace ingredients might be in your afternoon snack.

If someone is maintaining a healthy body weight with the occasional vending machine snack or diet soda thrown in, that person is much healthier than the person who's still 40-pounds overweight and worrying about GMOs and artificial sweeteners. This book is meant to help you finally make a lasting change and not get caught up in the minor details. Worry about those little things later.

The truth is that the most effective diet is the one you can stick to for a long time. Making a lasting change takes time, and bouncing from diet to diet, losing and gaining the same 5 pounds over and over, isn't going to get you anywhere. If having a cookie every night after dinner helps you finally reach your goal weight, that's significantly better than trying to cut out all sweets and resorting to binge eating every weekend, making no long-term progress.

How Much Is Too Much?

Now that you know that it's okay to eat fun foods regularly, you need to understand how much of your diet should consist of these treats. The big concern here is overall internal health, not pure weight loss or weight gain.

Micronutrients are vital for internal health. Heart health, bone health, mental health, energy levels, your mood... all of these things, and many more rely on adequate nutrition. These micronutrients come from fruits, vegetables, lean meats, healthy fats, and other things that would typically be considered healthy foods.

The issue then with eating processed foods is that they are generally lacking in these micronutrients. Spending your macros on processed foods means you'll have fewer available for whole foods that provide those good nutrients. Many people try to use a multivitamin or greens supplement as nutritional insurance, which isn't a bad idea, but nothing will be as good as eating whole foods every day.

A good rule is to follow the 80/20 rule. 80 percent of the time, try to eat whole, unprocessed foods. These are the foods that supply the nutrition you need to feel your best. The other 20 percent of the time, have some fun. Think of a few treats you love and figure out how to work them into your meal plan. You can do a small treat every day or eat whole foods most of the week and have one or two fun meals. The choice is yours. Just keep in mind that the more processed foods you eat, the greater risk you have of feeling less optimal, as you're lowering your nutrient intake.

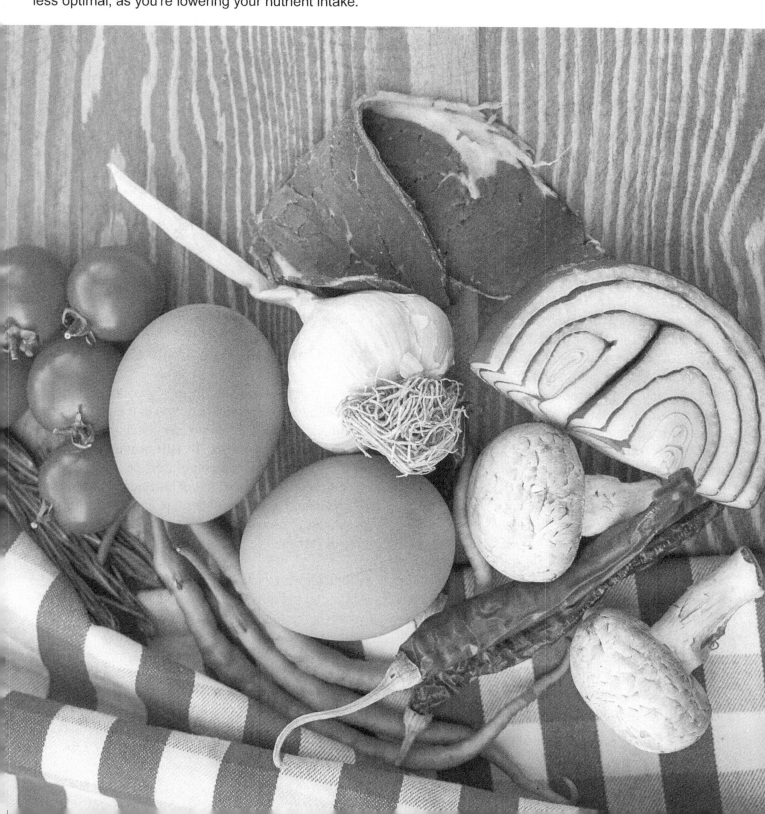

Chapter 4: How to Calculate Macros

This chapter teaches you how to calculate how many macros you should be consuming each day for your body and fitness goals. This will provide a clear path to achieve those goals and establish long-term healthy eating patterns.

The 5 Steps to Macro Success

There are five key steps to help you find success with the macro diet:

- Decide your goal
- Calculate your daily calories
- Calculate your daily macros
- Plan for success
- Track your daily numbers.

1. Decide Your Goal

Creating a specific, measurable, achievable, relevant, and time-framed (SMART) goal will help keep you focused. For example, if your goal is "to lose weight," that's not specific enough. A better approach to this would be: "In three months, I want to be 8 pounds lighter. I will track my macros to ensure I'm meeting my protein-energy requirements, weigh myself monthly, and use the fitting of my jeans to monitor my progress."

- Losing Weight: You probably have heard of the "3,500-calorie rule." That is, to lose 1 pound of fat in a week, one must burn 500 calories or eat 500 calories less every day for the week (3,500 calories total). With this approach, one technically should lose around 20 pounds in 5 months, right? Unfortunately, that's not necessarily the case. It doesn't take into account that our bodies differ in metabolic rate and genetics. So, although this approach may work in the short term, it's important to recognize that weight loss is not straightforward or linear, and adjustments will need to be made to your overall intake.

-

- Exercise: There are no hard-and-fast rules around exercising to lose weight while tracking your macros; however, healthy eating, combined with the consistent physical activity, does support a more sustainable lifestyle change. To maintain a healthy body weight, build strength, and reduce your risk of disease, the Canadian Physical Activity Guidelines recommend healthy adults from 18 to 64 get a minimum of 150 minutes of moderate to vigorous aerobic activity weekly and muscle-bone strengthening activities twice weekly. Examples of moderate-intensity physical activity include brisk walking and bike riding. Examples of vigorous activity would be jogging and cross-country skiing. Muscle-strengthening activities include push-ups, sit-ups, lifting weights, and climbing stairs.

- Gaining Lean Muscle: The macro diet is also a popular way of eating to build muscle. This is because it gives you control over how much energy you are consuming each day—especially when it comes to energy from protein—so that you can consume a surplus of calories required to add weight and grow muscle.

- Maintaining Good Health: The macro diet is not just for weight loss or gain—it's also ideal for maintaining your health in the long run.

2. Calculate Your Daily Calories

Now that you've decided on your goal, let's figure out how many calories you need. You can calculate this manually using the following calculations or use an online calculator like "**NIDDK.NIH.gov/bwp.**", "**If It Fits Your Macros calculator**" or "**Katy Hearn Fit calculator**". The benefit of calculating manually is that you gain a deeper understanding of how factors, such as age and physical activity, impact your overall energy needs.

- Find Out How Much Energy You Use at Rest: You first need to know your basal metabolic rate (BMR), which is the number of calories your body uses at rest each day to sustain basic functioning.

To begin, you need to know what your height and weight are in metric units. Divide your weight in pounds by 2.2 and round it up or down to the nearest whole figure to find out the kilograms. Then multiply your height in inches (1 foot = 12 inches) by 2.54

and round it up or down to calculate the centimeters. Make note of these figures. Next, fill out the calculation for your sex below, taking into account your weight, height, and age:

BMR MALE: (10 X WEIGHT IN KG) + (6.25 X HEIGHT IN CM) − (5 X AGE) + 5 =

BMR FEMALE: (10 X WEIGHT IN KG) + (6.25 X HEIGHT IN CM) − (5 X AGE) − 161 =

So, your BRM x your activity factor (from above) = your TDEE _____

This number is a fairly accurate measurement of the average total energy your body burns every day.

- How It Looks in Real Life: To make more sense of the above numbers, let's see how they add up for a real person. For example, Jane is a 30-year-old moderately active woman who weighs 165 pounds and is 5 foot 4 inches tall, which equals 64 inches. Dividing her weight in pounds by 2.2, she writes down that she is 75 kilograms. Multiplying her height in inches by 2.54, she notes that she is 163 centimeters tall.

She can figure out her BMR using the formula for women:

(10 X 75) + (6.25 X 163) − (5 X 30) − 161 =

750 + 1,019 − 150 − 161 = 1,458 CALORIES

(HER BMR: THE MINIMUM AMOUNT OF ENERGY HER BODY NEEDS.)

TDEE = BMR X MODERATELY ACTIVE FACTOR

= 1,458 X 1.55 = 2,260 CALORIES

(THE DAILY AMOUNT OF ENERGY SHE NEEDS TO MAINTAIN HER WEIGHT.)

ADJUST CALORIES IF YOU WANT TO LOSE WEIGHT.

As a guideline, you can subtract 250 to 500 calories from your TDEE to find out how many calories you need to consume per day to lose weight.

TDEE − 500 CALORIES = CALORIES TO CONSUME EACH DAY FOR WEIGHT LOSS

For Jane, this would be 2,260 − 500 = 1,760 calories.

I really do believe caloric intake should not be less than 1,400 calories per day. Anything lower makes it difficult to consume essential nutrients, and as a comparison, 1,200 calories is what a sedentary seven-year-old child should be consuming. The goal is "healthy" weight loss with a flexible eating pattern. Instead of over-restriction, consume enough nutrient-dense foods and adjust your lifestyle to burn more calories.

- ADJUST CALORIES IF YOU WANT TO GAIN MUSCLE: To gain muscle, add 250 to 500 calories to your TDEE. This should be done in conjunction with a strength training exercise.

- **Calculate Your Daily Macros**

Now that you know how many calories you need to lose weight, it's easy to figure out how many grams of each macronutrient you need to eat daily. The calculations are not absolute. It's a framework built around an average weekly macronutrient ratio that provides adequate intakes of essential nutrients; you may decide you prefer a different macro intake because of your needs or tastes. This is fine, so long as you consume enough food to satisfy what is known as the acceptable macronutrient distribution ranges (AMDR).

As per the 2015–2020 Dietary Guidelines for Americans, AMDR for people's daily intake of calories is 45% to 65% carbohydrates, 10% to 35% protein, and 20% to 35% fat. Eating within these ranges is vital to support tissue growth, facilitate energy production, and prevent disease-related to nutritional deficiency. The meal plan in this book uses the average weekly macro ratio of 45% carbohydrates, 30% protein, and 25% fat for both weight loss and weight maintenance. Using an average ratio accommodates the 80/20 rule, which allows you to eat a varied diet.

If You Want to Lose or Maintain Weight: Let's start with calculating the grams of macros to consume each day if you want to lose weight. Remember:

- Carbohydrates provide 4 calories per gram and will make up 45% of total daily calories.

- Protein provides 4 calories per gram and will make up 30% of total daily calories.

- Fat provides 9 calories per gram and will make up 25% of total daily calories.

Let's calculate Jane's macros. She needs 1,760 calories per day for weight loss.

JANE'S NEEDS									
MACRONUTRIENT	MACRONUTRIENT RATIO		DAILY CALORIE NEEDS		CALORIES PER MACRONUTRIENT		CALORIES PER GRAM		DAILY MACRONUTRIENT GRAMS
CARBOHYDRATES	0.45	x	1760	=	792	÷	4	=	198
PROTEIN	0.30	x	1760	=	528	÷	4	=	132
FAT	0.25	x	1760	=	440	÷	9	=	49

Jane's daily weight loss needs are:

1,760 Calories 198 g Carbs 132 g Protein 49 g Fat

YOUR NEEDS									
MACRONUTRIENT	MACRONUTRIENT RATIO		DAILY CALORIE NEEDS		CALORIES PER MACRONUTRIENT		CALORIES PER GRAM		DAILY MACRONUTRIENT GRAMS
CARBOHYDRATES	0.45	x	_____	=	_____	÷	4	=	_____
PROTEIN	0.30	x	_____	=	_____	÷	4	=	_____
FAT	0.25	x	_____	=	_____	÷	9	=	_____

Your daily weight loss needs are:

_____Calories _____g Carbs _____g Protein _____ g Fat

If You Want to Build Muscle: To build muscle, you can do the same calculations as above, but add 250 to 500 calories to your TDEE (rather than subtracting) and increase the ratio of protein you consume to promote muscle growth. A good starting point for this is 45% carbs, 35% protein, and 20% fat.

How Precisely Do I Need to Hit My Daily Targets? Eating exactly the right number of grams of any given macronutrient per day is easier said than done. For this reason, it's okay to leave some wiggle room from day to day, as long as across the week they average out close to your daily macro target and macro ratio.

Although there is no hard rule as to how much you can be outside of your macro ratio split, I recommend you do not consume more or less than 5% of a particular macro in your ratio split. If you continuously are above or below this range, it's a good indication that you need to adjust your targeted macronutrient ratio to meet this need.

3. Plan for Success

It's often said that failing to plan is planning to fail. Given the importance of hitting your daily macro targets to achieve results, you will need to plan your nutrition ahead of time.

Beyond the first 14 days, you should plan your weekly eating schedule. Think about what an average day looks like to you and write down how many meals you eat. Next, attempt to evenly split your macros across each meal. If your goal is 120 grams of protein per day, and you eat three meals, you'd want to aim for 40 grams for each meal. This groundwork makes hitting your macros much more manageable rather than trying to get all of one type of macro in one sitting. Once you have a general split, you can scale macro allotments up or down for different times of the day.

Once you have this, it is important to plan your shopping, food prep, and cooking to save time putting together meals to avoid scrambling to find the right foods at the last minute. Here are some useful tips to help you throughout the week:

• Set aside some time every week to plan your meals and create a grocery list.

• Check to see what foods you have on hand before doing your shopping.

• Batch-cook for multiple days so that you have meals already prepared.

• Find meals that you love to eat that fit your macro profile and cook those frequently.

4. Track Your Daily Numbers

For any new skill, you need to practice before you become good at it. Understanding and tracking macros is no different. If you don't know what or how much to eat, you may feel so overwhelmed that you feel like throwing in the towel by eating whatever is in front of you. Remember, although it may seem detail-oriented at first, this is a short-term approach until you have a better understanding of the macro content of different foods. Eventually, it'll become second nature, and you won't need to track.

Chapter 5: Workout Plan

A weight loss plan is incomplete without exercise, especially for the endomorph body type. Exercise allows you to reduce fat and increase metabolism. Cardiovascular exercises, including running, will help you burn calories. You have to burn more calories than your consumption. Make sure to burn extra fat.

As per ACE (American Council on Exercise), people should follow a well-rounded exercise. You have to focus on strength training and cardiovascular activities. See these examples:

HIIT (High-Intensity Interval Training): In HIIT, you have to alternate between different periods of low intensity and high-intensity exercise, along with rest. You can do this exercise 2–3 times per week. Each session must be 30 minutes long.

SST (Steady State Training): These may be long sessions of low to moderate-intensity exercise. Some suitable SST exercises are swimming, jogging, and walking. If you have an endomorph body type, you can follow SST for almost 30 to 60 minutes three times a week.

Weight and Strength Training Exercises

If you want to build muscles, you can follow strength training exercises. It must be an important part of your weight loss plan.

A healthy muscle group is necessary to increase metabolism because muscle tissues can burn calories. They help your body in using fat for fuel. Several exercises and weight training routines are useful. Experts recommend several compound exercises. With the help of compound exercises, you can use different units and body tissues. It offers the best control of your body. You can use body weight, barbell, and free weights during exercise.

Here is a list of exercises and a 2-week workout plan to get the most of your Macro Diet. Each workout consists of multi-joint, upper body, lower body, core, and mobility exercises. A combination of these exercises ensures you receive a full-body workout.

Week 1—Day 1

Total Workout Time: 30 minutes

Exercise	Reps	Sets	Rest
Air Squats	10–15	2	90 seconds
Tricep Dips	10–15	2	90 seconds
Swimmers	10–15	2	90 seconds
Glute Bridge	10–15	2	90 seconds
Press Ups	10–15	2	90 seconds
Dead Bug	10–15	2	90 seconds
Standing Toe Touches	10–15	2	90 seconds
Cow	30 seconds	2	90 seconds

How to Do the Exercises

1. Air Squats

Air squats are a multi-joint exercise working your leg muscles, including the glutes, quads, hamstrings, calves, and core. Squatting is needed for a range of everyday tasks, from standing up from your chair to picking something up off the floor.

Instructions:

1. To perform the air squat, stand with your feet shoulder-width apart.
2. Push your hips back and bend the knees until your buttocks are lower than your knees.
3. Keep your back straight, and your core engaged throughout the exercise.
4. Drive through your midfoot to return to standing.
5. During extension, push your knees out.

Tip: When setting up for the air squat, "screw" your feet into the floor.

Easier Option: Lower your buttocks ¼ of the way down, rather than below your hips.

Harder Option: Add weight or add a jump during extension.

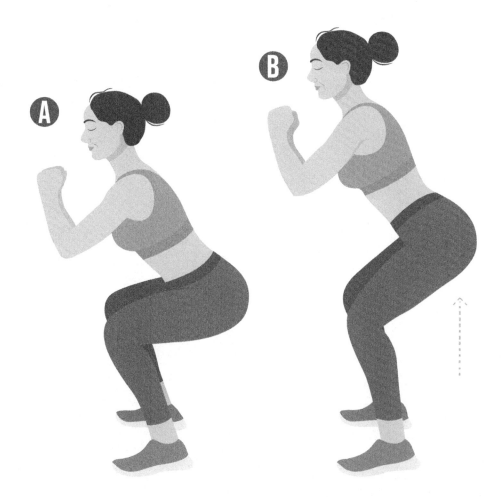

2. Tricep Dips

Tricep dips are an upper body exercise focusing on the backs of your arms. Our triceps help us extend our arms.

Instructions:

1. To perform a tricep dip, you'll need a raised surface such as a chair or a bench.

2. Edge your buttocks just off the side of the surface so your feet are flat on the floor.

3. Bend your elbows until they form a 90-degree angle, then push through your palm to return to extension.

Tip: Look forward rather than down at your feet to keep your neck in a neutral position.

Easier Option: Bring your feet closer to the elevated surface.

Harder Option: Move your feet further from the elevated surface.

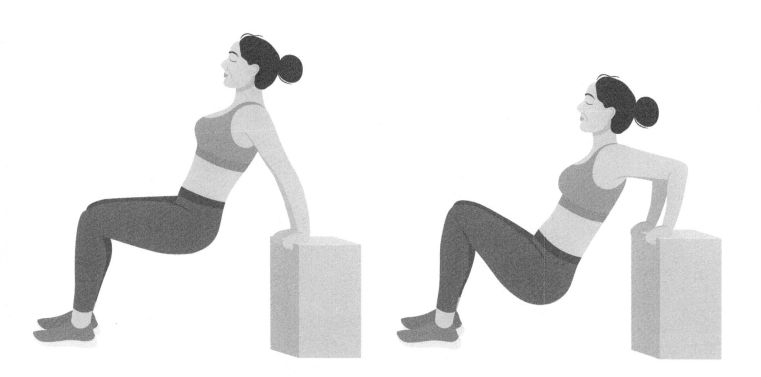

3. Swimmers

Swimmers are an advanced version of alternating superman. They work single limb strength and stability in your upper back, lower back, glutes, hamstrings, and core. It's a great exercise for improving posture and alleviating back pain.

Instructions:

1. Begin lying face down with your legs extended and arms above your head.

2. Push your hips into the floor while squeezing your core and buttocks.

3. Lift your arms and feet off the floor slightly; this is your starting position.

4. Lift your right arm and left foot as far as you comfortably can.

5. Lower to the starting position while simultaneously lifting your left arm and right foot.

Tip: Think of the action like a front crawl.

Easier Option: Perform alternating superman.

Harder Option: Hold a weight in each hand.

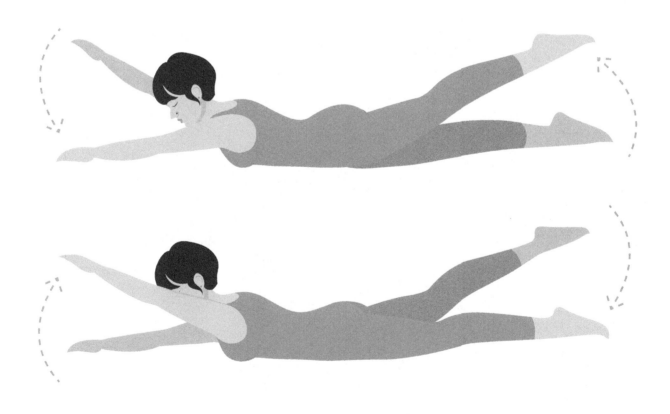

4. Glute Bridge

The glute bridge works the glutes, core, lower back, hamstrings, and hips. The glute bridge can also be used to alleviate knee and lower back pain.

Instructions:

1. Begin lying on the floor with your legs extended and arms at your side.

2. Pull your feet to your buttocks until they are flat on the floor.

3. Push your shoulders, upper back, and lower back into the floor while squeezing your core.

4. Engage your glutes, then push your hips towards the sky.

5. At the top of the movement, your knees, hips, and shoulders should be aligned.

6. Pause at the top for two seconds before slowly lowering.

Tip: Push your knees out during extension.

Easier Option: Place your feet further from your core.

Harder Option: Place a weight on your groin area

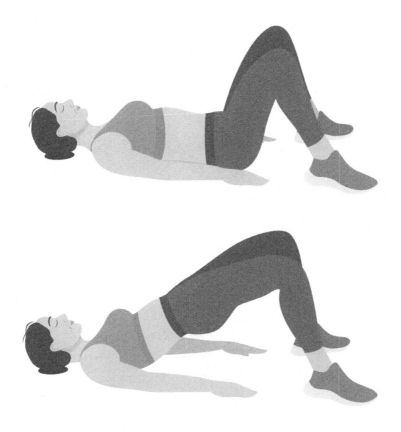

5. Press Up

The press-up is one of the best body weight exercises for building upper body pushing strength. It helps in building strength in the chest, shoulders, triceps, biceps, and back. It also helps in strengthening the shoulder joint.

Instructions:

1. Start in the plank position.

2. Place your hands under your shoulders and your toes on the floor.

3. Your shoulders, buttocks, and ankles should all be aligned.

4. Squeeze your core and buttocks.

5. Bend the elbows to lower your chest to the floor.

6. Pause for one second before pushing through the palms to return to the starting position.

Tip: Your hips and shoulders should move together. Don't bend your back to make the movement easier.

Easier Option: Perform the press-ups on your knees.

Harder Option: Pause for 4 seconds at the bottom of the press-up.

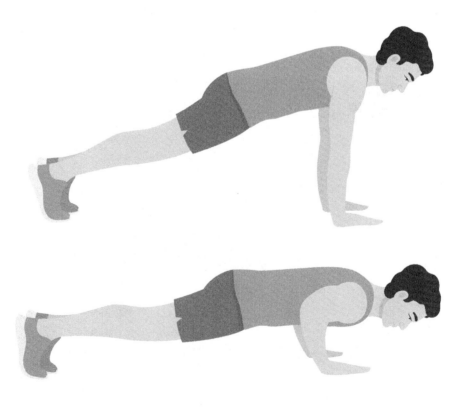

6. Dead Bug

Dead bugs are a core exercise to help develop your core strength, coordination, and balance. They're great for strengthening the smaller muscles in your shoulders and hips too.

Instructions:

1. To perform the dead bug, begin by lying face-up on a mat.

2. Bring your knees towards your chest at a 90-degree angle and extend your arms towards the ceiling.

3. Slowly lower your right arm and left leg towards the floor.

4. Stop about 1-inch above the floor, pause for a second, and then return to the center before repeating on the other side.

Tip: Press your lower back into the floor to engage your core.

Easier Option: Only move your leg or arm, not both.

Harder Option: Hold a weight in your hands.

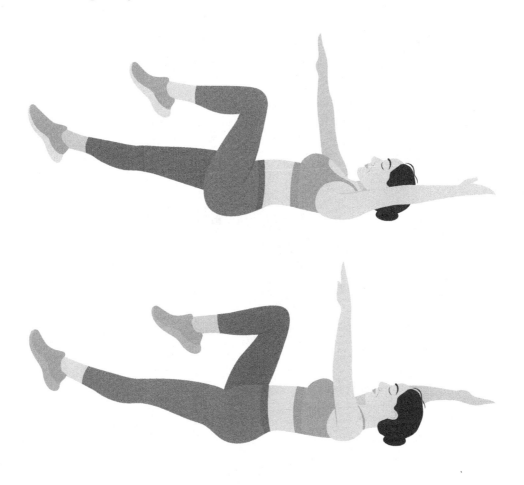

7. **Standing Toe Touches**

Standing toe touches are a great exercise to improve your mobility, core, and leg strength. It predominantly works your obliques and hamstrings.

Instructions:

1. Stand tall with your feet shoulder-width apart.

2. Keeping your legs straight, raise your right leg in front of you as far as you comfortably can.

3. Meanwhile, raise your left arm to meet the toe.

4. Slowly lower and repeat on your opposite side.

Tip: Keep your core and glutes tight.

Easier Option: Bend your knees slightly.

Harder Option: Hold a weight in each hand.

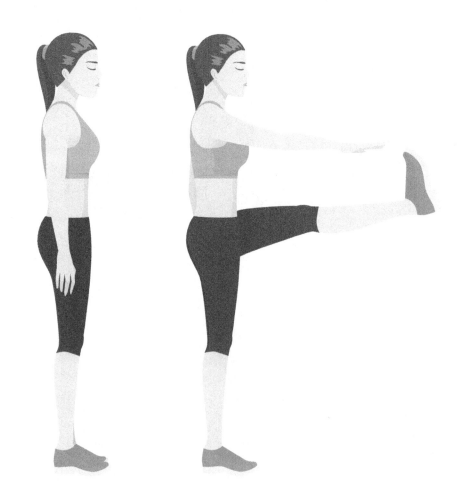

8. Cow

The cow is a yoga pose that stretches your torso and neck. It's a great way to improve your posture and spine health.

Instructions:

1. Begin on your hands and knees.

2. Ensure your hands are directly under your shoulders and knees under your hips.

3. Keep your head in a neutral position and squeeze your core.

4. Lift your chest while drawing the belly button down. Hold this position.

Tip: Pull your shoulder blades apart and down.

Easier Option: Release the position every 10 seconds.

Harder Option: Perform the cat-cow exercise.

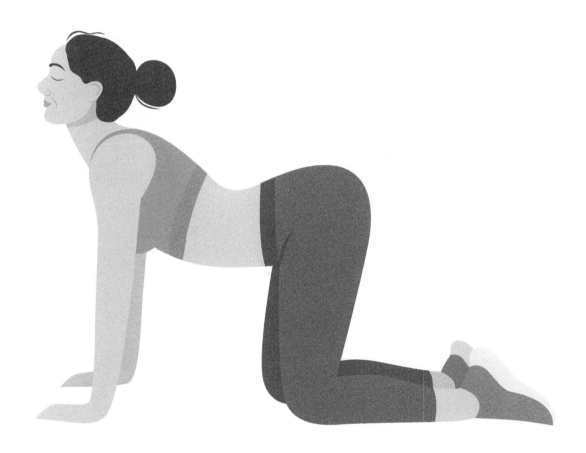

Week 1—Day 2

Total Workout Time: 30 minutes

Exercise	Reps	Sets	Rest
Deadlift	10–15	2	90 seconds
Bird Dog Plank	10–15	2	90 seconds
Clams	10–15	2	90 seconds
Hollow Archs	10–15	2	90 seconds
Long Lunge	10–15	2	90 seconds
Hammer Curl	10–15	2	90 seconds
Calf Raises	10–15	2	90 seconds
Boat	30 seconds	2	90 seconds

How to Do the Exercises

9. Deadlift

The deadlift is one of the best exercises for building full-body strength. The deadlift primarily trains the muscles in your legs, lower back, and core. It is also a great exercise to improve your posture. During the deadlift, you need to engage your shoulders, spine, and hips. This crosses over into good posture.

Instructions:

1. Begin standing tall with your feet hip-width apart.
2. Hold a weight in each hand at your sides.
3. Pull your shoulder blades together and engage your core.
4. Send your hips back, then bend at the knees.
5. Lower the weight as far as you can without rounding your back.
6. When you've reached maximal depth, push the hips forward to return to standing.

Tip: Keep your neck in a neutral position by looking at a spot on the floor in front of you.

Easier Option: Perform the exercise without weights.

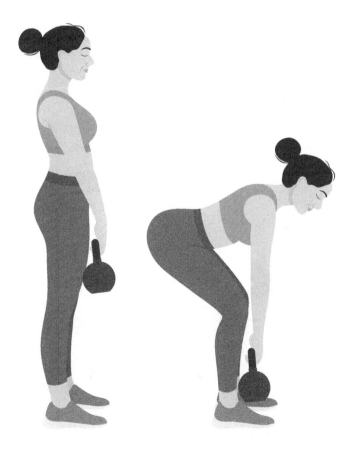

10. Bird Dog Plank

The bird dog plank improves full-body stability and strengthens your spine, back, core, glutes, hamstrings, shoulders, and triceps. Transferring your weight onto single limbs is a great way to build joint strength and control.

Instructions:

1. Start in the plank position.
2. Place your hands under your shoulders and toes on the floor.
3. Your shoulders, buttocks, and ankles should all be aligned.
4. Squeeze your core and buttocks.
5. Extend your right leg and left arm until they are parallel to the floor.
6. Hold for two seconds before returning to the starting position.
7. Repeat on the opposite side.

Tip: Practice shifting your weight onto your arms before getting your legs involved.

Easier Option: Raise your legs only.

Harder Option: Hold for 5 seconds at the top of the movement.

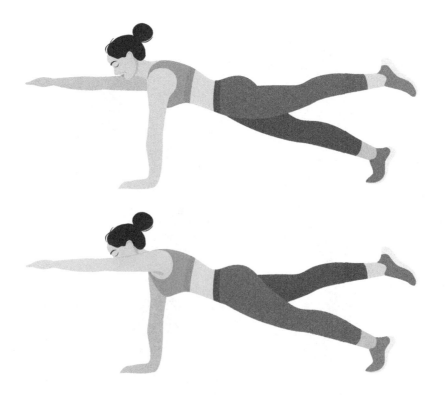

11. Clams

Clams build strength in the glutes as well as the inner and outer thighs. Your glutes play a significant role in stabilizing your pelvis; therefore, we must keep it strong.

Instructions:

1. Begin lying on your left side with your hips and shoulders aligned.

2. Bend your knees slightly and prop your head up with your hand.

3. Brace your core and tuck your belly button in.

4. Keeping your toes together, rotate your right knee as far as you can without breaking hip alignment.

5. Pause for two seconds before returning to the starting position.

Tip: Keep your neck still.

Easier Option: Reduce the range of motion.

Harder Option: Wrap a resistance band just above your knees.

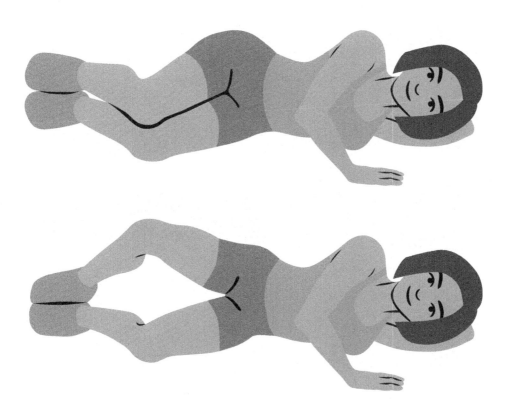

12. Hollow Archs

Hollow archs help build a strong and stable core. They target the abdominals, diaphragm, hip flexors, and core. They **are** also beneficial **for** improving your posture.

Instructions:

1. Begin lying on the floor with your legs extended and your arms above your head.

2. Push your shoulders, upper back, and lower back into the floor while squeezing your core.

3. Squeeze your ankles together and bring your arms to your ears.

4. Lift your upper back and feet off the floor until you feel that your abs tense.

5. Hold for a second before slowly lowering.

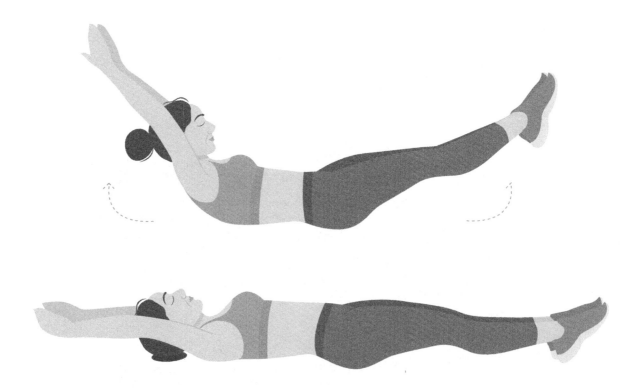

13. Long Lunge

The long lunge is a quad-dominant exercise developing single-leg strength and stability. The long lunge targets your quadriceps, thighs, hips, and glutes.

Instructions:

1. Begin standing tall with your feet shoulder-width apart.

2. Take a long step forward with your right foot while keeping your left foot planted.

3. Bend your right leg until it creates a 90-degree angle at the knee.

4. Ensure your shoulders are relaxed and your core is engaged.

5. Repeat the exercise on your opposite leg.

Tip: Keep your pelvis neutral, your chest high, and your back straight.

Easier Option: Feel free to cut back on the range of motion and stay above a 90-degree angle.

Harder Option: Hold weights at your side or wear a weighted backpack.

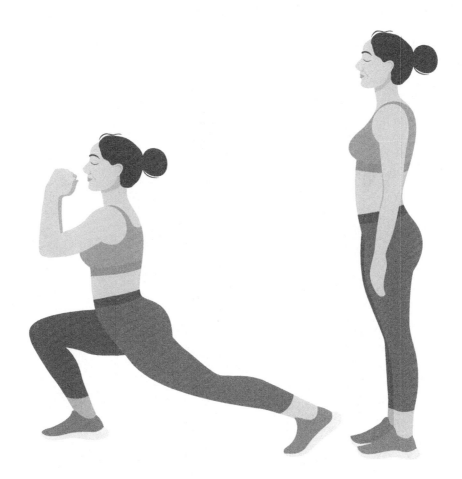

14. Calf Raises

Calf raises build strength in the lower legs. Lower leg strength is vital for protecting your ankles from injury.

Instructions:

1. Stand tall with your feet just inside shoulder-width.
2. Point your toes forward.
3. Hold a weight in each hand.
4. Squeeze your shoulder blades together.
5. Push through the balls of the feet, raising your heels above your toes.
6. Hold for two seconds before slowly lowering.
7. Repeat this movement.

Tip: Place your toes on an elevated surface, such as a book, to increase the range of motion.

Easier Option: Perform the exercise without weights.

Harder Option: Do not let your feet touch the floor between reps. Keep tension in your lower leg by pausing half an inch from the floor.

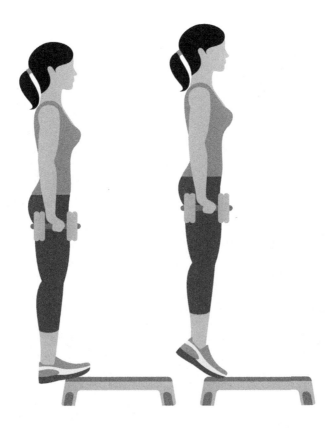

15. Boat

The boat pose develops core strength and stability in the back and abdomen. Specifically, it strengthens the abdominals, hip flexors, and spine.

Instructions:

1. Begin seated with your knees bent and your feet flat on the floor.

2. Place your hands next to your hips.

3. Keeping your back straight, lean your torso back while lifting your feet off the floor.

4. Extend your legs and push your chest up.

5. Extend your arms forwards off the floor while maintaining a tight core. (Your body should now be in a V-shape.)

6. Hold this position.

Tip: Spread your shoulder blades apart.

Easier Option: Bend your knees and keep your hands on the floor.

Harder Option: Lower your feet to an inch off the floor, then raise them back up to work the lower abdomen harder.

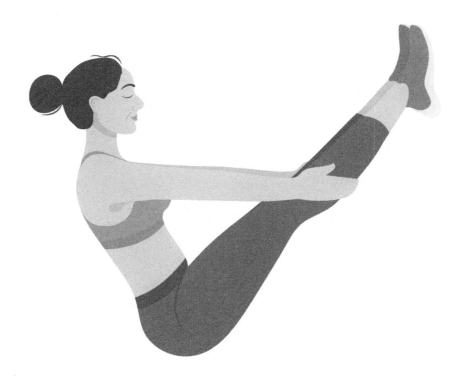

Week 1—Day 3

Total Workout Time: 30 minutes

Exercise	Reps	Sets	Rest
Plié Squat	10–15	2	90 seconds
Split Stance Row	10–15	2	90 seconds
Donkey Kicks	10–15	2	90 seconds
Leg Raises	10–15	2	90 seconds
Single-Leg Box Squat	10–15	2	90 seconds
Shoulder Press	10–15	2	90 seconds
Reverse Lunges	10–15	2	90 seconds
Sphinx	30 seconds	2	90 seconds

16. Plié Squat

The plié squat strengthens the quads, hamstrings, glutes, and calves while increasing the range of motion in your hips.

Instructions:

1. Stand with your feet outside shoulder-width apart.
2. Rotate your feet out to a 45-degree angle.
3. Put your hands on your hips.
4. Keep your back straight and your core engaged throughout.
5. Drive through your midfoot to return to standing.
6. During extension, push your knees out.

Tip: Keep your chest up.

Easier Option: Perform a wide squat.

Harder Option: Place a resistance band just above your knees.

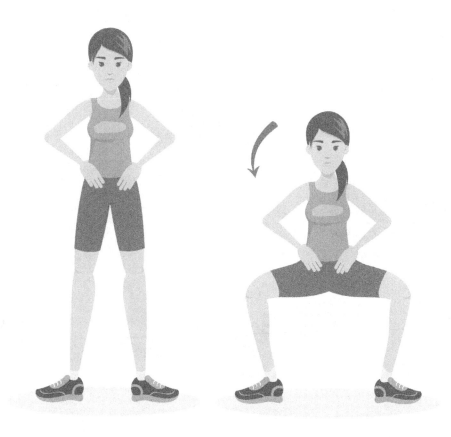

17. Split Stance Row

The split stance position improves your core and leg stability and strength. The rowing portion of the exercise works your shoulders, back, biceps, and triceps.

Instructions:

1. Stand tall with your feet shoulder-width apart and a weight in your right hand.
2. Step your left leg in front of you and your right leg behind; this is your split stance position.
3. Bend your left knee slightly, then lean your torso until it's close to parallel to the floor.
4. Engage your core and buttocks.
5. Bend your right elbow to pull the weight to your chest.
6. Pause for one second, then slowly lower to full extension.
7. Perform half the repetitions on your right side and the other half on your left.

Tip: Place your left hand on your left thigh for stability.

Easier Option: Perform the exercise without weights.

Harder Option: Pause for 4 seconds at the top of the movement.

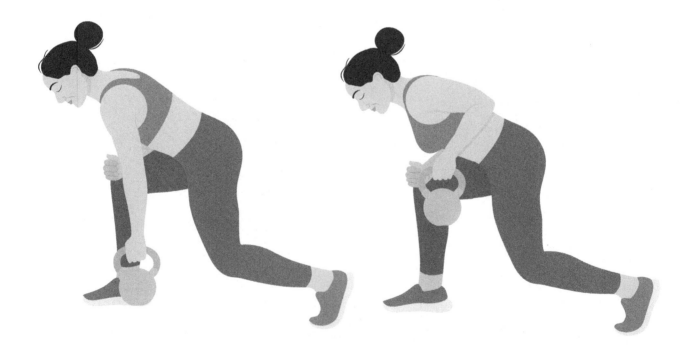

18. Donkey Kicks

Donkey kicks work your core and glute muscles to build strength and stability.

Instructions:

1. Start on your hands and knees.
2. Your hands should be directly under your shoulders and your knees under your hips.
3. Keep your back flat, core engaged, and glutes tensed.
4. Keeping your leg bent, raise your right leg until your thigh is in line with your torso.
5. Pause for one second before lowering to the starting position.
6. Repeat the movement on your left leg.

Tip: Keep your hips squared. Avoid any torso rotation.

Easier Option: Reduce the range of motion.

Harder Option: Place a resistance band above your knees.

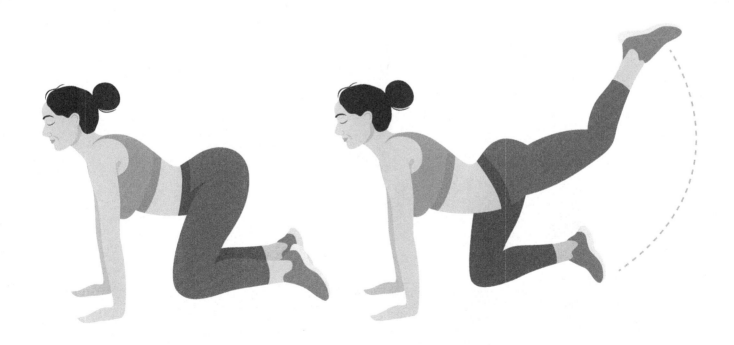

19. Leg Raises

Leg raises build your core strength and stability. Leg raises focus on the lower part of your abdominals, which can be difficult to target.

Instructions:

1. Begin lying on the floor with your legs extended and arms at your side.

2. Push your shoulders, upper back, and lower back into the floor while squeezing your core.

3. Squeeze your ankles together.

4. Lift your feet off the floor to a 90-degree angle.

5. Hold for one second before slowly lowering.

Tip: Control the movement, don't rely on momentum.

Easier Option: Bend your legs to a 90-degree angle.

Harder Option: Do not lower your legs to the floor. Pause 1 inch from the floor before performing the next repetition.

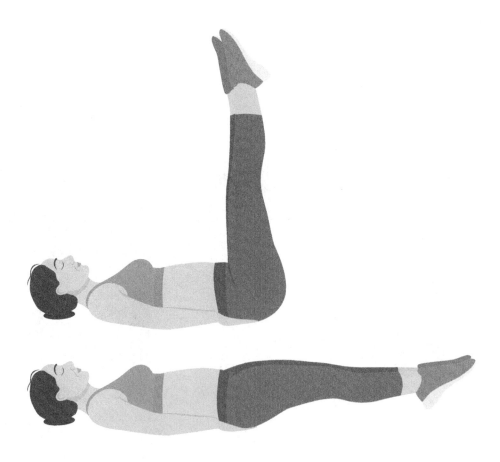

20. Single-Leg Box Squat

Single leg box squats are similar to bench squats, but focus on single-limb movement. Single limb movements help eliminate any muscle imbalances. The single-leg box squat develops strength in your glutes, hamstrings, and quads. This is a great crossover to real-life movements, such as standing up out of a chair. If you don't have a box, use a raised surface of similar height, such as a chair, bench, or low wall.

Instructions:

1. To perform the single-leg box squat, stand with feet shoulder-width apart.
2. Squeeze your shoulder blades, core, and buttocks.
3. Lift your right leg off the floor 1 inch or 2.
4. Send your hips back and bend your left knee until you are sitting on the bench.
5. After a brief pause, drive your hips up to return to standing while keeping your core tight and back neutral.
6. Perform half the repetitions on your left leg and half on your right.

Tip: It's important to pause on the box. This exercise aims to eliminate any rebound movement.

Easier Option: Perform regular bench squats.

Harder Option: Hold a weight at chest height.

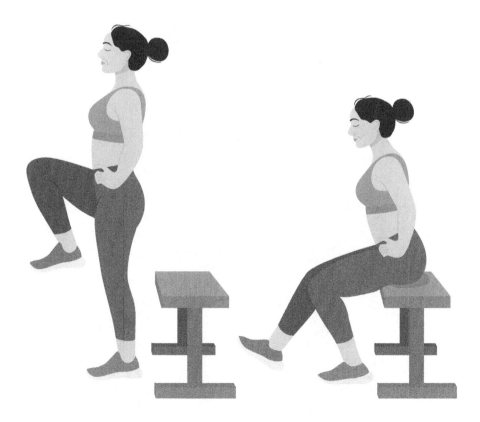

21. Shoulder Press

The shoulder press strengthens your shoulders and upper back. It's an excellent crossover for overhead press movement, such as putting your bag into overhead storage.

Instructions:

1. Stand tall with your feet hip-width apart with a weight in each hand.

2. Bend the elbows to bring the weights to your shoulders; this is your starting position.

3. Pull your shoulder back, engage your core, and squeeze your buttocks.

4. Push the weights towards the sky until they reach full extension.

5. Pause for one second, then lower the weights back to the starting position.

Tip: Push your head forward during extension.

Easier Option: Perform the exercise without weights.

Harder Option: Perform the exercise on the floor with your legs extended and your torso upright.

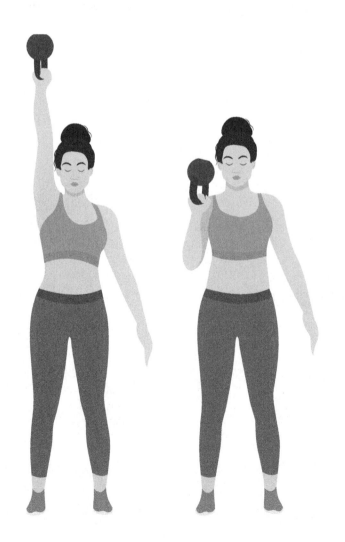

22. Reverse Lunges

Reverse lunges are a core, glute, and hamstring-focused exercise. Unlike regular lunges, we will be stepping back with our legs to initiate the movement rather than stepping forward. This places less stress on your joints and gives you more stability in your front leg. Therefore, it's a great exercise for those with knee problems, balance issues, or restricted hip mobility.

Instructions:

1. Begin standing with your feet hip-width apart.

2. Take a long step back with your right leg and bend your left knee until it reaches a 90-degree angle.

3. Keep your core and buttocks tight.

4. Drive through the midfoot of your left leg to return to standing.

5. During the extension, push your left knee out to the side.

6. Repeat on the opposite side.

Tip: Focus on a specific place on the wall throughout the exercise to help with your balance.

Easier Option: Reduce the range of motion by staying above a 90-degree angle.

Harder Option: Hold a weight in each hand.

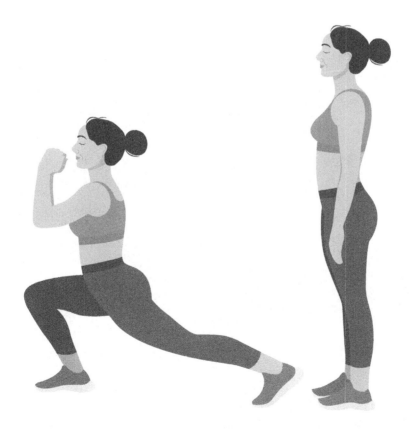

23. Sphinx

The sphinx strengthens your spine and glutes while stretching the chest, shoulders, and abdominals.

Instructions:

1. Begin lying face-down on the floor.
2. Place your elbows under your shoulders and place your feet hip-width apart.
3. Push your feet and quads into the floor.
4. Push through your elbows to raise your chest and head.
5. Keep your hips on the floor and pull your shoulder blades together.
6. Hold this position.

Tip: Rotate your thighs inwards.

Easier Option: Place a rolled-up towel in a U-shape on the floor. Lie on the towel to support the lift.

Harder Option: Extend your arms fully.

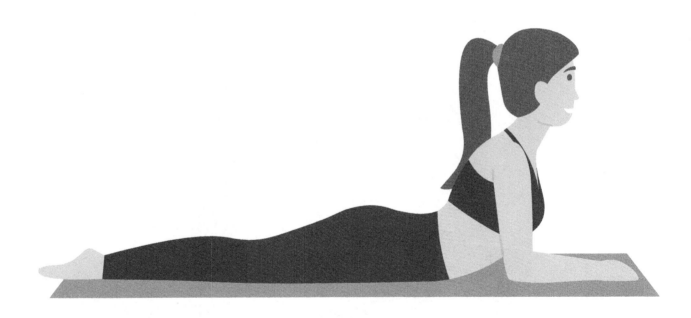

Week 2—Day 1

Total Workout Time: 30 minutes

Exercise	Reps	Sets	Rest
Single-Leg Raise	10–15	2	90 seconds
Lateral Raises	10–15	2	90 seconds
Side Lunges	10–15	2	90 seconds
Cat Cow	10–15	2	90 seconds
Knee to Elbow Extension	10–15	2	90 seconds
Shrugs	10–15	2	90 seconds
Wide Squat	10–15	2	90 seconds
Cobra	30 seconds	2	90 seconds

How to Do the Exercises

24. Single-Leg Raise

Single-leg raises are an advanced version of plank hip dips. They develop full-body strength and stability. The additional hip raise also puts more emphasis on the glutes.

Instructions:

1. Begin sitting on the floor with your legs extended and your torso upright.
2. Place your hands on the floor behind your shoulders.
3. Lean back so your arms take the weight of your body.
4. Bring your feet to your buttocks while remaining flat on the floor.
5. Push through your feet and palms to lift your hips slightly off the floor.
6. From here, fully extend your left leg towards the sky.
7. Lift your hip and extend your arms.
8. Pause for one second, then lower back to the floor.
9. Perform half the repetitions on your right leg and half on your left.

Tip: Push through your foot on the floor to assist the lift.

Easier Option: Keep both feet on the floor.

Harder Option: Place a resistance band just above your knees.

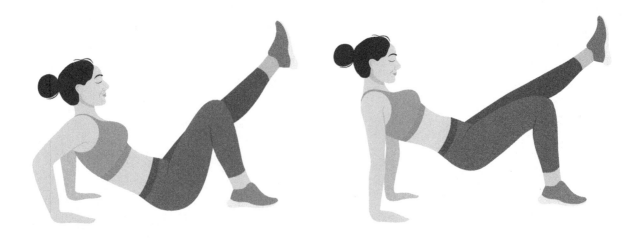

25. Lateral Raises

Lateral raises focus on building your shoulder strength, specifically your lateral shoulder strength. They also help strengthen the shoulder joint.

Instructions:

1. Stand tall with your feet hip-width apart and a weight in each hand at your sides.

2. Pull your shoulders back, squeeze your buttocks, and engage your core.

3. Slightly bend your elbows, then lift the weight out to the side until your arms are parallel to the floor.

4. Pause for one second, then slowly lower back to the center.

Tip: Initiate the movement with your elbows.

Easier Option: Perform the exercise without the weights.

Harder Option: Reduce the range of motion to keep tension in the shoulders.

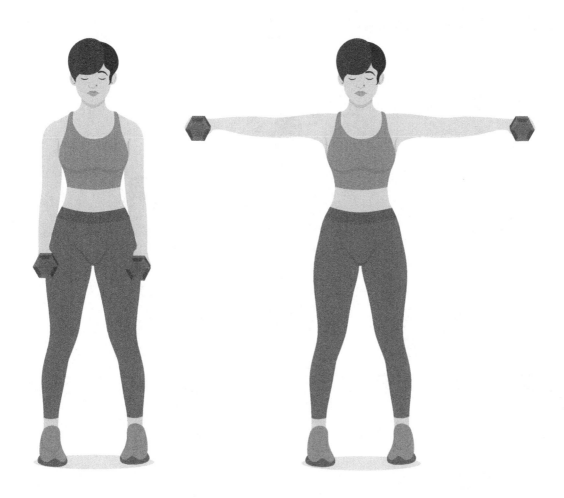

26. Side Lunges

Side lunges help improve your balance, strength, and stability. They work your inner and outer thighs, also known as your adductors and abductors. The sideways movement helps prepare your body for side-to-side movements, such as shuffling during sports play.

Instructions:

1. Stand tall with your feet hip-width apart.

2. Take a wide step out to your right while bending your right knee as far as you can without rounding your back.

3. Keep both feet flat on the floor.

4. Push through your right foot to return to standing.

5. Repeat on your left side.

Tip: Point your knees in the same direction as your feet.

Easier Option: Step out to the side without bending your knee.

Harder Option: Hold a weight close to your chest.

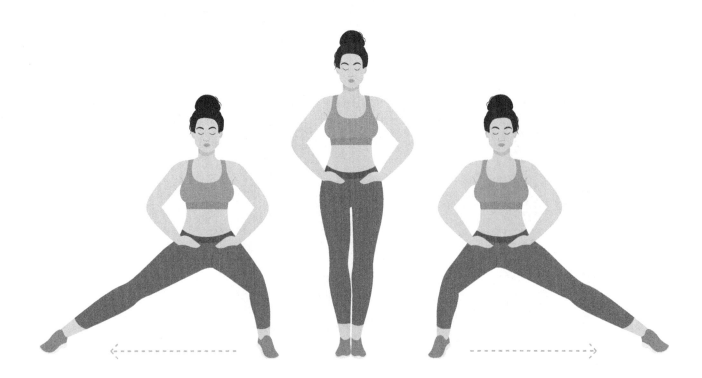

27. **Cat-Cow**

The cat-cow is a mobility exercise used to improve posture and balance. **It** also helps you relax while relieving stress.

Instructions:

1. Start on your hands and knees with your hips over your knees and your shoulders over your hands.

2. From here, lower your chest without bending your arms.

3. Then, bring your upper back up towards the ceiling, rounding your shoulders.

Tip: Imagine a piece of string is attached to your chest, and someone is pulling it towards the floor and ceiling.

Easier Option: Perform the movement in a chair.

Harder Option: Work through the 2 positions in one fluid movement.

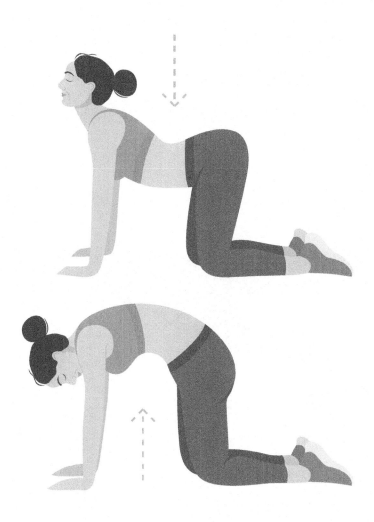

28. Knee to Elbow Extension

Knee to elbow extensions are similar to mountain climbers, but focus more on the glutes. They also work your shoulders, hamstrings, quads, triceps, and core.

Instructions:

1. Begin in a press-up position with your arms and legs fully extended.

2. Your weight should be spread between your hands and feet.

3. Keep your shoulders, hips, and feet aligned throughout the movement, as well as keeping your core engaged.

4. Bring your right knee towards your right elbow.

5. Drive your right foot back and raise your foot to the sky.

6. Pause for a second before returning to the starting position.

7. Repeat the movement on your left leg.

Tip: Lift your leg until you feel that your glute contracts fully.

Easier Option: Only perform the leg lift; do not bring your knee to your elbow.

Harder Option: Place a resistance band just above your knees.

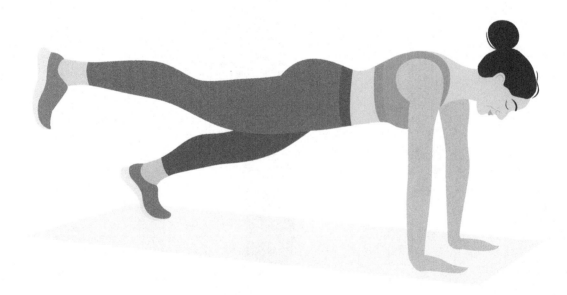

29. Shrugs

Shrugs build strength in your shoulders, neck, and upper back. They also help in reducing neck and shoulder strain, as well as in improving posture.

Instructions:

1. Stand tall with your feet hip-width apart.

2. Hold a weight in each hand at your sides.

3. Rotate your palms into your body.

4. Squeeze your core and buttocks, and draw your shoulder blades back.

5. Keeping your arms straight, lift your shoulders as high as possible.

6. Pause for one second before lowering to the starting position.

Tip: Imagine you are trying to touch your ears with your shoulders.

Easier Option: Perform the exercise without weights.

Harder Option: Perform the exercise with a barbell.

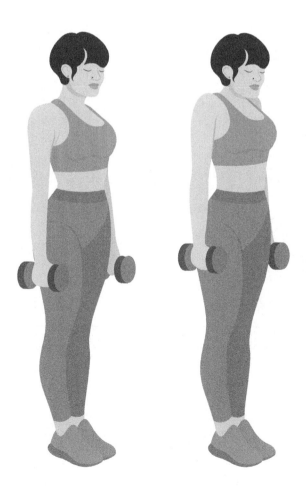

30. Wide Squat

Wide squats require more hip extension than regular air squats. Therefore, it places more emphasis on hip strength. However, just like normal air squats, wide squats work your glutes, quads, hamstrings, calves, and core.

Instructions:

1. To perform the wide squat, stand with your feet outside shoulder-width apart.
2. Push your hips back and bend your knees until your buttocks are just above knee height.
3. Keep your back straight and your core engaged throughout the exercise.
4. Drive through your midfoot to return to standing.
5. During the extension, push your knees out.

Tip: Initiate the movement from your hips, not your knees.

Easier Option: Bring your feet closer together to perform a regular air squat.

Harder Option: Hold a weight at chest height, or wear a weighted backpack.

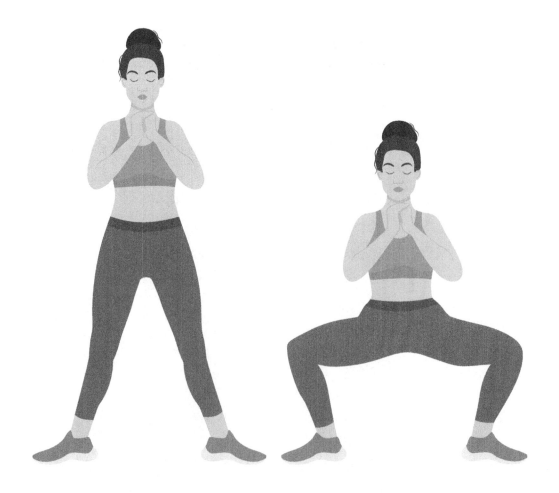

31. **Cobra**

The cobra improves your posture and alleviates back pain by strengthening the shoulders, arms, and back muscles.

Instructions:

1. Begin lying face-down on the floor.
2. Place your hands by your ribs and place your feet hip-width apart.
3. Push your feet and quads into the floor.
4. Push through your palms to raise your chest and head.
5. Keep your hips on the floor and pull your shoulder blades together.
6. Hold this position.

Tip: Keep a slight bend in your arms.

Easier Option: Place your forearms on the floor and don't extend your arms fully.

Harder Option: Rest your feet on a book or block to extend the stretch.

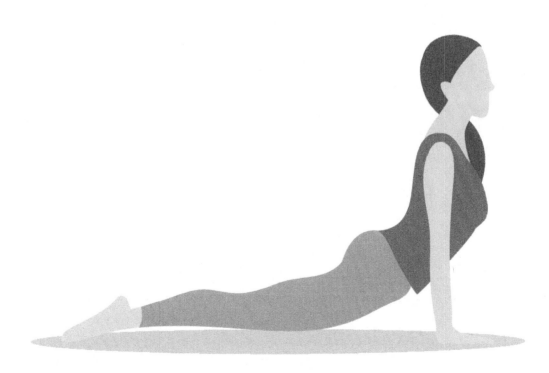

Week 2—Day 2

Total Workout Time: 30 minutes

Exercise	Reps	Sets	Rest
Kneeling Shoulder Press	10–15	2	90 seconds
Bicep Curl	10–15	2	90 seconds
Bench Squats	10–15	2	90 seconds
Bicycle Crunches	10–15	2	90 seconds
High Knees	10–15	2	90 seconds
Single Arm Row	10–15	2	90 seconds
Leg Abduction	10–15	2	90 seconds
Crescent Lunge	30 seconds	2	90 seconds

How to Do the Exercises

32. Kneeling Shoulder Press

The kneeling shoulder press is an excellent exercise for building the upper body and core strength. Similar to a regular shoulder press, but the kneeling position provides instability, which forces your core to work.

Instructions:

1. Stand tall with your feet hip-width apart and a weight in your right hand.
2. Bend your right arm to bring the weight to your shoulder.
3. Take a long step forward with your left leg, lowering the hips until your right knee touched the floor.
4. Squeeze your core and buttocks tight.
5. Push the weight above your head to full extension at the elbow.
6. Pause for a second, then slowly lower your back to your shoulder.
7. Repeat half the reps on your right arm before switching to your left side.

Tip: Place your opposite hand on your hip to remain balanced.

Easier Option: Perform the exercise without weights.

Harder Option: Perform the exercise with a weight in each hand.

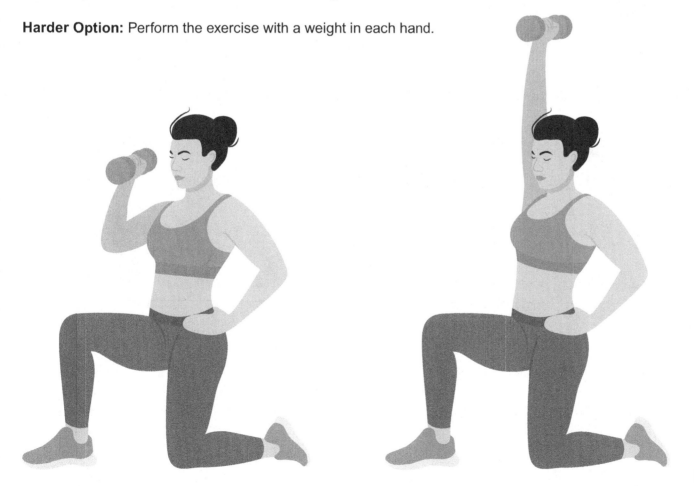

33. Bench Squats

Instructions:

1. To perform the bench squat, stand with your feet shoulder-width apart.

2. Squeeze your shoulder blades, core, and buttocks.

3. Send your hips back and bend your knees until you are sitting on the bench.

4. After a brief pause, drive your hips up to return to standing while keeping your core tight and your back neutral.

Tip: It's important to pause on the bench. This exercise aims to eliminate any rebound movement.

Easier Option: Use your hands to assist you up off the bench.

Harder Option: Hold a weight at chest height.

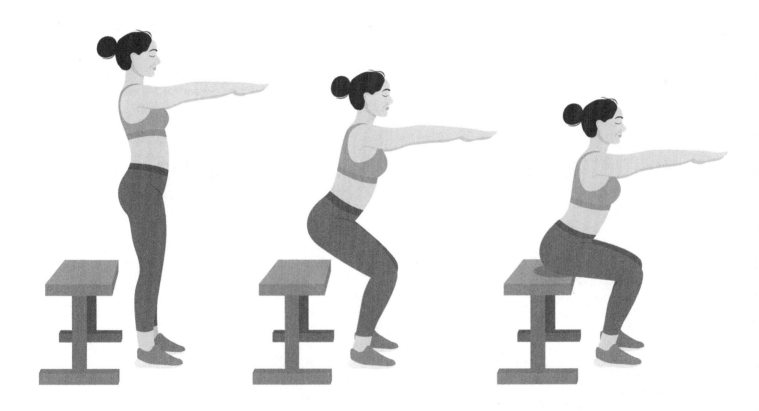

34. Bicycle Crunches

Bicycle crunches are predominantly a core exercise focusing on rotational strength. A strong core protects the spine and helps you perform better in everyday tasks. The extension of the legs also activates the hip muscles.

Instructions:

1. Start lying face-up on the floor with your legs fully extended.

2. Lift your feet off the floor until they are over your hips at a 90-degree angle.

3. Place your fingers on your temples and raise your upper back off the floor. This is your starting position.

4. Move your right elbow towards your left knee while simultaneously extending your right leg.

5. Return your arms and legs to the starting position before repeating the movement on the opposite side.

Tip: Do not pull your neck up.

Easier Option: Keep your upper back on the floor.

Harder Option: At the top of the movement, when your knee and elbow are touching, pause for two seconds.

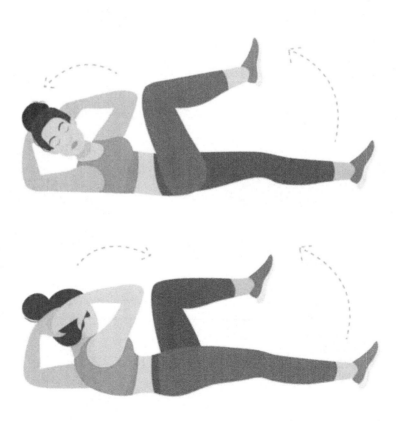

35. High Knees

High knees will ramp up your heart rate while working the glutes, quads, hamstrings, core, and calves. High knees cross over well to running, so it will prepare you for when you need to run for the bus or chase your grandchildren around the garden.

Instructions:

1. Start with your feet hip-width apart.//
2. Raise your right knee up to your chest, then lower it back to the floor.
3. Repeat this movement on your left leg.
4. When you get comfortable, simultaneously drive up one leg while lowering the other—just like you're running.

Tip: Put your hands straight out in front of your chest. Aim to hit your palms with your knee on each rep.

Easier Option: Try to bring your knees up to hip height or as high as comfortable.

Harder Option: Use your arms to replicate a sprinting motion.

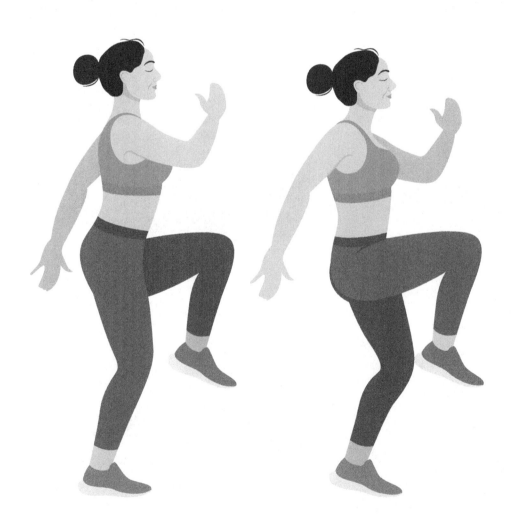

36. Single Arm Row

The single-arm row builds pulling strength in your shoulders, upper back, and core. Everyday tasks rely on pulling actions, such as opening a cupboard or door.

Instructions:

1. Hold a weight in your right hand.
2. Place your left hand and left knee on the side of a bench.
3. Your knee should be directly under your hips and your hand under your shoulder.
4. Draw the shoulder blades back while squeezing the glutes and core.
5. Keeping your back straight, bend your right elbow to bring the weight to your chest.
6. Pause for one second before slowly returning to extension.
7. Perform half the repetitions on your right side and half on the left.

Tip: Do not rotate the torso. Ensure all movement comes from the arm.

Easier Option: Perform the exercise without weight.

Harder Option: Pause for three seconds at the top of the movement.

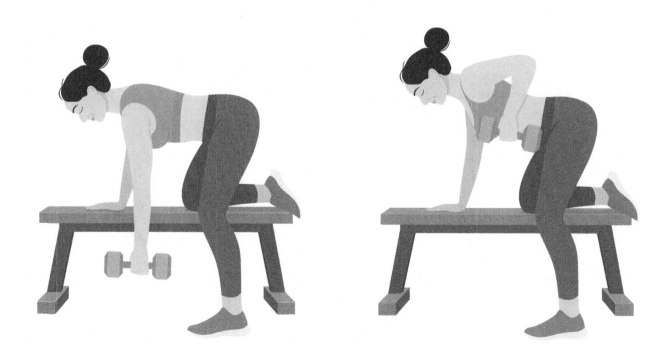

37. Leg Abduction

Leg abduction is a common everyday movement. We perform abduction when we step to the side or get out of bed. **Leg** abductions strengthen the **hips** and glutes.

Instructions:

1. Begin lying on your right side with your legs extended and your right arm propping your torso up.

2. Squeeze your core and buttocks.

3. Hold for two seconds before slowly lowering.

4. Perform half the repetitions on your left leg and half on your right.

Tip: Keep your hips square.

Easier Option: Slightly bend your legs.

Harder Option: Place a resistance band just above your knees.

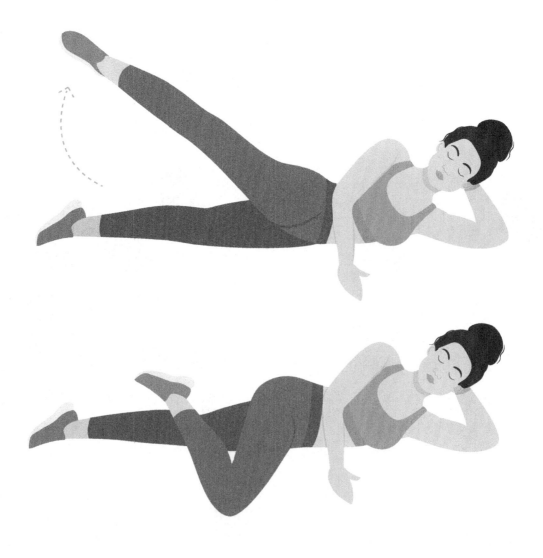

38. Crescent Lunge

The crescent lunge improves flexibility in your hips, groin, and shoulders.

Instructions:

1. Begin standing tall with your feet shoulder-width apart.
2. Take a long step forward with your right foot while keeping your left foot planted.
3. Bend your right leg until it creates a 90-degree angle at the knee.
4. Ensure your shoulders are relaxed and your core is engaged.
5. Lower your hips and rest your back leg on the floor.
6. Extend your arm above your head and lean back.
7. Hold this position before repeating on the opposite leg.

Tip: Keep your hips square and pushed towards the floor.

Easier Option: Place a towel or block under your back foot.

Harder Option: Hold a weight in each hand

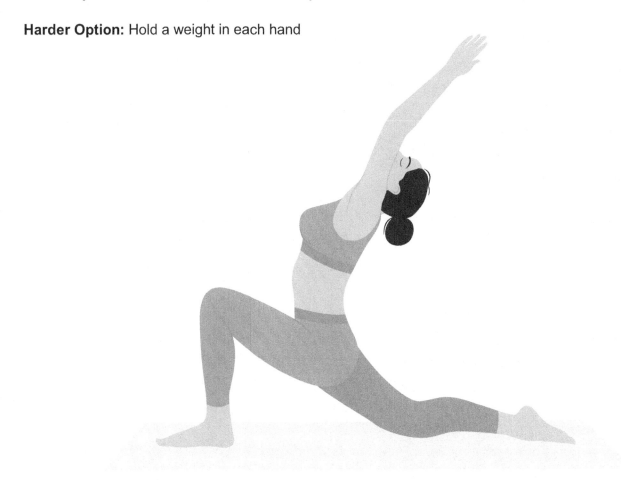

Week 2—Day 3

Total Workout Time: 30 minutes

Exercise	Reps	Sets	Rest
Plank Hops	10–15	2	90 seconds
Front Raises	10–15	2	90 seconds
Knee to Chest	10–15	2	90 seconds
Flutter Kicks	10–15	2	90 seconds
Mountain Climbers	10–15	2	90 seconds
Plank Toe Taps	10–15	2	90 seconds
Jumping Jacks	10–15	2	90 seconds
Baby Cobra	30 seconds	2	90 seconds

How to Do the Exercises

39. Plank Hops

Plank hops strengthen your core and cardiovascular system. They also help in building strength in the shoulders, glutes, quads, hamstrings, and triceps.

Instructions:

1. Start in the plank position.

2. Place your hands under your shoulders and your toes on the floor.

3. Your shoulders, buttocks, and ankles should all be aligned.

4. Squeeze your core and buttocks.

5. Jump your feet to land below your buttocks.

6. Briefly pause before jumping back to the plank position.

Tip: Keep your feet together.

Easier Option: Step each leg in rather than jump.

Harder Option: Rebound the jumps without pausing between them.

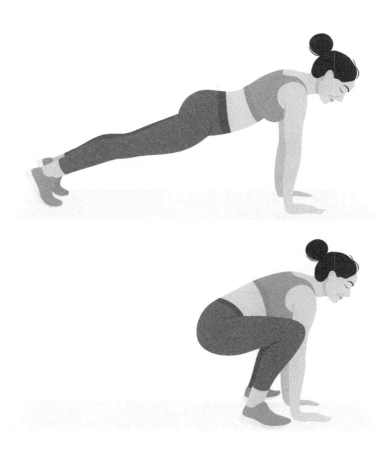

40. Front Raises

Front raises focus on building your shoulder strength, specifically your anterior shoulder strength. They also help strengthen the shoulder joint.

Instructions:

1. Stand tall with your feet hip-width apart and a weight in each hand at your sides.

2. Pull your shoulders back, squeeze your buttocks, and engage your core.

3. Slightly bend your elbows, then lift the weight out in front of you until your arms are parallel to the floor.

4. Pause for one second, then slowly lower back to the center.

Tip: Keep your wrists tight; don't let them get sloppy.

Easier Option: Perform the exercise without the weights.

Harder Option: Slow down the movement by counting to three during the lowering phase.

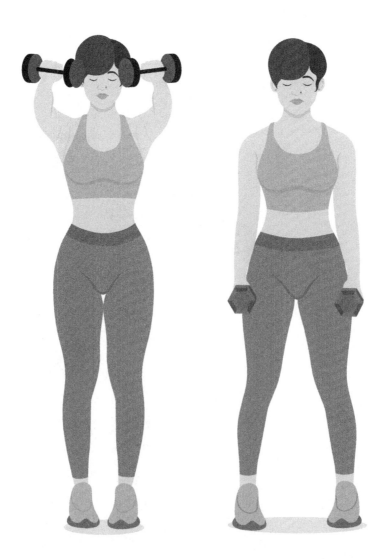

41. Knee to Chest

Knee to chests improves your mobility, core, and leg strength. They work your hip flexors, abdominals, and quads.

Instructions:

1. Stand tall with your feet shoulder-width apart.

2. Squeeze your core and glutes while pulling your shoulder blades together.

3. Bring your right knee to your chest, hold briefly, and then lower.

4. Repeat on your left leg.

Tip: Look at a spot on the floor to help you balance.

Easier Option: Perform the movement seated.

Harder Option: Hold at the top of the movement for four seconds.

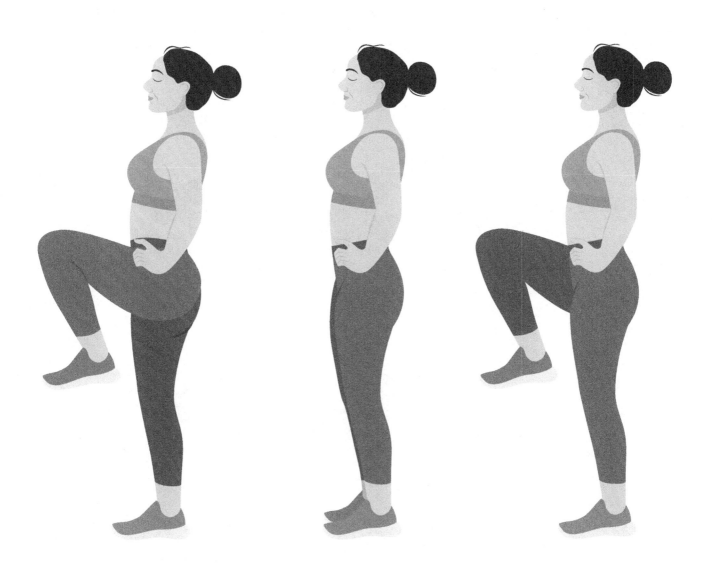

42. Flutter Kicks

Flutter kicks strengthen your core by targeting the lower abdominal and hip flexors.

Instructions:

1. Begin lying on the floor with your legs extended and your arms at your side.

2. Push your shoulders, upper back, and lower back into the floor while squeezing your core.

3. Lift your feet 5-inches off the floor while keeping your lower back pressed into the floor.

4. Cross your feet over each other—like a scissor action.

Tip: Control the movement; don't be tempted to go fast.

Easier Option: Raise your feet higher.

Harder Option: Lift your upper back off the floor during the movement.

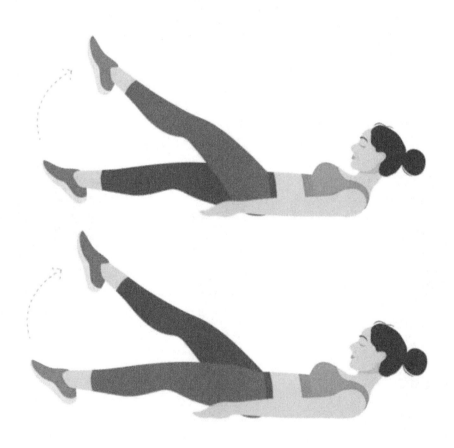

43. Mountain Climbers

Mountain climbers build your cardiovascular fitness, full-body strength, and agility. Mountain climbers place specific emphasis on the shoulders, hamstrings, quads, triceps, and core.

Instructions:

1. Begin in a press-up position with your arms and legs fully extended.

2. Your weight should be spread between your hands and feet.

3. Keep your shoulders, hips, and feet aligned throughout the movement, as well as keeping your core engaged.

4. Bring your right knee towards your right elbow.

5. Drive your right foot back to the starting position while simultaneously bringing your left knee to your chest.

Tip: Keep your neck in a neutral position. Prevent your chin from tucking in or looking to the sky.

Easier Option: Eliminate moving your legs simultaneously. Instead, bring your knee to your elbow and back again before repeating the movement on your opposite leg.

Harder Option: Instead of driving your knee to your elbow, place your foot just outside your hand. A greater range of motion will enhance your flexibility as well as strength.

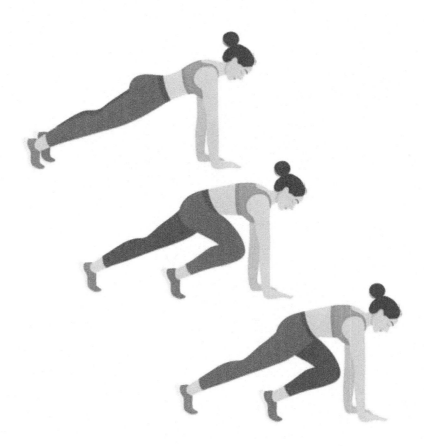

44. Plank Toe Taps

The plank improves full-body stability and strengthens your spine, back, core, glutes, hamstrings, shoulders, and triceps. Plank toe taps place greater emphasis on the abdominals and obliques, as well as helping to improve hip mobility.

Instructions:

1. Start in the plank position.

2. Place your hands under your shoulders and your toes on the floor. (Your shoulders, buttocks, and ankles should all be aligned.)

3. Squeeze your core and buttocks.

4. Lift your hips towards the sky and touch your left foot with your right hand. (Your feet and left hand should stay in place.)

5. Continue alternating.

Tip: Be careful not to drop your hips too low during the descent.

Easier Option: Move your hands as close to your toes as possible.

Harder Option: Do not alternate. Perform half the repetitions on one side before completing the other half on the opposite side.

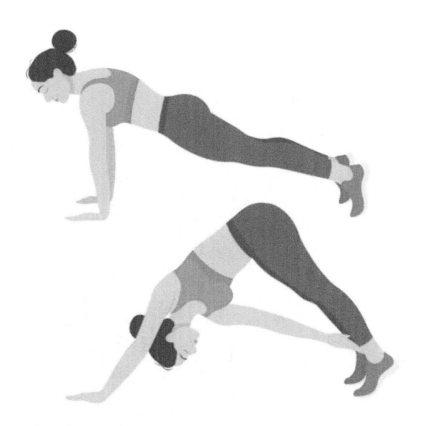

45. Jumping Jacks

Jumping jacks are a total-body exercise specifically focusing on your hips, lower back, thighs, shoulders, and hamstrings. They are also great for building bone strength and improving cardiovascular fitness.

Instructions:

1. Stand with your feet shoulder-width apart, then jump into the air while moving your arms and legs away from your body.

2. You should land in a star shape with your arms and legs extended.

3. Jump back into the air while bringing your arms and legs back to the body.

Tip: Keep your eyes facing forward to help you balance.

Easier Option: Step out to the side instead of jumping.

Harder Option: Begin by touching your toes, then extending into the star shape.

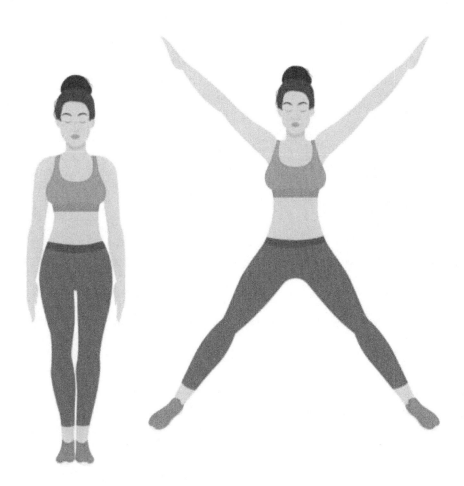

46. Baby Cobra

The baby cobra is a modified version of the cobra pose. It improves your posture and alleviates back pain by strengthening the shoulders, arms, and back muscles.

Instructions:

1. Begin laying face-down on the floor.
2. Place your hands by your ribs and place your feet hip-width apart.
3. Push your feet and quads into the floor.
4. Keep your hips on the floor and pull your shoulder blades together.
5. Hold this position.

Tip: Your arms should not extend. Focus on stretching your shoulder blades rather than creating movement.

Easier Option: Hold the same position but do not force your shoulder blades to move.

Harder Option: Perform the full cobra.

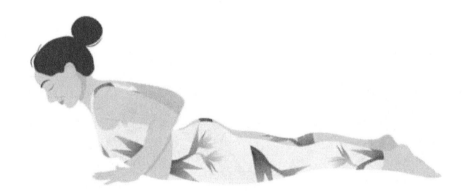

Chapter 6: Foods to Eat and Avoid During Macro Diet

Food Items to Eat on a Macro Diet

If you have a mesomorphic or ectomorphic body try to eat as naturally as possible, I'll write down a list of the food you should choose more often:

- Seafood
- Low carb veggies
- Cheese
- Avocado
- Meat and Poultry
- Eggs
- Nuts and Seeds
- Coconut oil
- Olive oil
- Greek yogurt
- Cottage cheese
- Berries
- Shirataki noodles
- Olives

With an endomorphic body, you will need a particular fitness plan to shed pounds. The endomorphic fitness type is suitable for your body. As per the theory of this diet, endomorphs have a slow metabolism. You may not be able to burn calories like mesomorphs and ectomorphs. Extra calories can be converted into fats. Moreover, you do not have sufficient tolerance for carbohydrates.

The best diet for your body may have a high protein and fat intake. It may be similar to a paleo diet. Remember, the diet may help you lose fat while improving the energy of your body. Some excellent sources of proteins and fats are:

- Olive oil
- Macadamia nuts
- Beef
- Fatty fish
- Egg yolk
- Walnuts
- Cheese

There is no need to avoid carbohydrates. Carbs offer sufficient energy to your body. By removing carbohydrates from your meals, you may feel fatigued and sluggish. Moreover, extremely low carbohydrates in your diet may increase the chances of gastrointestinal issues. For this reason, choose complex carbohydrates, such as vegetables. Starchy vegetables, such as tubers, potatoes, whole grains, fruits, and legumes, are good sources of complex carbs.

You must not consume simple carbohydrates. These foods have high calories and sugar that may increase the chances of fat storage. Simple carbohydrates have white bread, cookies, cakes, pasta, and white rice.

The fruit is essential for the Macro Diet. If you are carb-sensitive, eat fruits at a moderate amount. In your meals, you can consider 35% fat, 35% protein, and 30% carbohydrates. Portion control plays an important role in decreasing body fat. It will help you to decrease calorie consumption. Try to eat almost 200–500 fewer calories than you usually consume. In this way, you can shed pounds and reach a weight loss goal.

Polyunsaturated and Monounsaturated Fats

The list includes:

- Dairy (low-fat) products, including cheeses, yogurt, and low-fat milk

- Poultry, including turkey and chicken

- Several nontropical vegetable oils, such as avocado oil, canola, and olive

- Different fish types, particularly fatty fish

- Eggs and egg whites

- Nontropcial nuts, such as walnuts, hazelnuts, and almonds

Your body needs sufficient carbohydrates. Here are some good examples to fit in your Macro Diet:

- Fruits (avoid pineapple and melons)

- Legumes and dried beans, including chickpeas, lentils, and kidney beans

- Whole wheat and whole-grain products, including whole-wheat bread and all-bran cereal

- Non-starchy veggies, including celery, cauliflower, and broccoli

- Starchy vegetables, including carrots, corn, yams, and sweet potatoes. Unrefined starchy veggies, including amaranth and quinoa.

Food Items to Avoid During a Macro Diet

Remember, insulin hormone helps blood sugars move in cells. For a Macro Diet, you have to avoid or limit carbohydrate-dense foods, including sugar and white flour.

Foods with carbohydrates can quickly release sugars into your bloodstream. As a result, you will notice dips and spikes in blood sugar. The body can turn sugars into fat instead of burning them to produce energy.

Therefore, people following this diet should avoid nutrient-poor and calorie-dense foods. Some food items are prohibited in the Macro Diet, such as:

- Bagels, traditional pasta, white rice, and white bread

- Sweets, chocolates, and candies

- Cakes and baked goods

- Sports drinks, energy drinks, and soft drinks

- Refined cereals, including puffed rice, instant oatmeal, and bran flakes

- Fried or processed foods

- Dairy products, including ice cream, whipped cream, and cream

- Red meats

- Alcohol

- Cooking oils with saturated fat, including coconut or palm oil

- Food with sodium

Chapter 7: Meal Plan

Week 1

Days	Breakfast	Lunch	Snack	Dinner
Day 1	Blueberry Fat Bombs	Slow Cooked Roasted Pork and Creamy Gravy	Keto Trail Mix	Baked Zucchini Noodles with Feta
Day 2	Cheesy Zucchini Triangles with Garlic Mayo Dip	Grilled Salmon and Zucchini with Mango Sauce	Cold Cuts and Cheese Pinwheels	Brussels Sprouts with Bacon
Day 3	Herbed Cheese Chips	Pot Roast with Green Beans	Zucchini Balls with Capers and Bacon	Bunless Burger—Keto Style
Day 4	Cauliflower Poppers	Garlic Chicken	Strawberry Fat Bombs	Coffee BBQ Pork Belly
Day 5	Crispy Parmesan Chips	Crispy Cuban Pork Roast	Kale Chips	Garlic & Thyme Lamb Chops
Day 6	Tex-Mex Queso Dip	Keto Barbecued Ribs	Roasted Radishes with Brown Butter Sauce	Jamaican Jerk Pork Roast
Day 7	Breakfast Roll-Ups	Turkey Burgers and Tomato Butter	Parmesan and Pork Rind Green Beans	Keto Meatballs

Week 2

Days	Breakfast	Lunch	Snack	Dinner
Day 1	Basic Opie Rolls	Keto Hamburger	Pesto Cauliflower Steaks	Mixed Vegetable Patties
Day 2	Bacon & Avocado Omelet	Chicken Wings and Blue Cheese Dressing	Tomato, Avocado, and Cucumber Salad	Roasted Leg of Lamb
Day 3	Bacon & Cheese Frittata	Salmon Burgers with Lemon Butter and Mash	Crunchy Pork Rind Zucchini Sticks	Salmon Pasta
Day 4	Bacon & Egg Breakfast Muffins	Cheesy Chicken Cauliflower	Cheese Chips and Guacamole	Skillet Fried Cod
Day 5	Bacon Hash	Chicken Soup	Cauliflower "Potato" Salad	Slow-Cooked Kalua Pork & Cabbage
Day 6	Bagels with Cheese	Chicken Avocado Salad	Loaded Cauliflower Mashed "Potatoes"	Steak Pinwheels
Day 7	Baked Apples	Chicken Broccoli Lunch	Keto Bread	Tangy Shrimp

Week 3

Days	Breakfast	Lunch	Snack	Dinner
Day 1	Tofu Mushrooms	Easy Meatballs	Cheese Stuffed Mushrooms	Beef & Broccoli Roast
Day 2	Onion Tofu	Chicken Casserole	Zucchini Tots	Grilled Pesto Salmon with Asparagus
Day 3	Spinach-Rich Ballet	Turkey and Cream Cheese Sauce	Avocado Yogurt Dip	Whole Chicken with Leek and Mushrooms
Day 4	Pepperoni Egg Omelet	Baked Salmon and Pesto	Keto Macadamia Hummus	Turkey and Leek Goulash
Day 5	Nut Porridge	Keto Chicken with Butter and Lemon	Easy & Perfect Meatballs	Salsa Turkey Cutlet and Zucchini Stir-Fry
Day 6	Parsley Soufflé	Salmon Skewers Wrapped with Prosciutto	Delicious Chicken Alfredo Dip	Fried Turkey and Pork Meatballs
Day 7	Bok Choy Samba	Buffalo Drumsticks and Chili Aioli	Eggplant Chips	Pepper, Cheese, and Sauerkraut Stuffed Chicken

Chapter 9. Breakfast Recipes

1. Blueberry Fat Bombs

Preparation time: 10 minutes | Cooking time: 0 minutes | Servings: 12

1/2 cup blueberries, mashed
1/2 cup coconut oil, at room temperature
1/2 cup cream cheese, at room temperature
A pinch of nutmeg
6 drops liquid stevia

1. Line 12-cup muffin tin with 12 paper liners.
2. Put all the ingredients and process until it has a thick and mousse-like consistency.
3. Pour the mixture into the 12 cups of the muffin tin. Put the muffin tin into the refrigerator to chill for 1 to 3 hours.

Calories: 120 | Fat: 12.5g | Fiber: 1.4g | Protein:3.1g Carbohydrates:2.1g

2. Cauliflower Poppers

Preparation time: 20 minutes | Cooking time: 30 minutes | Servings: 4

4 cups cauliflower florets
2 teaspoons olive oil
1/4 teaspoon chili powder
Pepper and salt

1. Preheat the oven to 450°F. Grease a roasting pan.
2. In a bowl, add all ingredients and toss to coat well.
3. Transfer the cauliflower mixture into a prepared roasting pan and spread in an even layer.
4. Roast for about 25–30 minutes.
5. Serve warm.

Calories: 102 | Fat: 8.5g | Fiber: 4.7g | Protein: 4.2g Carbohydrates:2.1g

3. Tex-Mex Queso Dip

Preparation time: 5 minutes | Cooking time: 10 minutes | Servings: 6

1/2 cup coconut milk
1/2 jalapeño pepper, seeded and diced
1 teaspoon minced garlic
1/2 teaspoon onion powder
1 ounce goat cheese
6 ounces sharp cheddar cheese, shredded
1/4 teaspoon cayenne pepper

1. Preheat a pot then add the coconut milk, jalapeño, garlic, and onion powder.
2. Simmer, then whisk in the goat cheese until smooth.
3. Add the cheddar cheese and cayenne and whisk until the dip is thick, for 30 seconds to 1 minute.

Calories: 149 | Fat: 12.1g | Fiber: 3.1g | Protein: 4.2g Carbohydrates:5.1g

4. Crispy Parmesan Chips

Preparation time: 10 minutes | Cooking time: 5 minutes | Servings: 8

1 teaspoon butter
8 ounces full-fat parmesan cheese,
shredded or freshly grated

1. Preheat the oven to 400°F.
2. Spread butter on a baking sheet.
3. The parmesan cheese must be spooned onto the greased baking sheet in mounds, spread evenly apart.
4. Spread out the mounds with the back of a spoon until they are flat.
5. Bake the crackers until the edges are browned, and the centers are still pale, for about 5 minutes.

Calories: 101 | Fat: 9.4g | Fiber: 3.1g | Protein: 1.2g Carbohydrates:2.5g

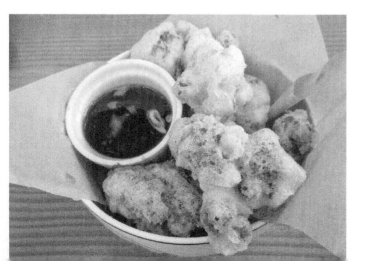

5. Cheesy Zucchini Triangles with Garlic Mayo Dip

Preparation time: 20 minutes | Cooking time: 30 minutes | Servings: 4

Garlic mayo dip:
- 1 cup crème fraiche
- 1/3 cup mayonnaise
- 1/4 teaspoon sugar-free maple syrup
- 1 garlic clove, pressed
- 1/2 teaspoon vinegar
- Salt and black pepper to taste

Cheesy zucchini triangles:
- 2 large zucchinis, grated
- 1 egg
- 1/4 cup almond flour
- 1/4 teaspoon paprika powder
- 3/4 teaspoon dried mixed herbs
- 1/4 teaspoon swerve sugar
- 1/2 cup grated mozzarella cheese

1. Start by making the dip: In a medium bowl, mix the crème fraiche, mayonnaise, maple syrup, garlic, vinegar, salt, and black pepper.
2. Cover the bowl with plastic wrap and refrigerate while you make the zucchinis.
3. Let the oven preheat at 400°F. And line a baking tray with greaseproof paper. Set aside.
4. Put the zucchinis in a cheesecloth and press out as much liquid as possible.
5. Pour the zucchinis into a bowl.
6. Add the egg, almond flour, paprika, dried mixed herbs, and swerve sugar.
7. Mix well and spread the mixture on the baking tray into a round pizza-like piece with 1-inch thickness.
8. Let it bake for 25 minutes.
9. Reduce the oven's heat to 350°F, take out the tray, and sprinkle the zucchini with the mozzarella cheese.
10. Let it melt in the oven.
11. Remove afterward, set aside to cool for 5 minutes, and then slice the snacks into triangles.
12. Serve immediately with the garlic mayo dip.

Calories: 286 | Fat: 11.4g | Fiber: 8.4g | Protein: 10.1g Carbohydrates: 4.3g

6. Herbed Cheese Chips

Preparation time: 15 minutes | Cooking time: 15 minutes | Servings: 8

- 3 tablespoons coconut flour
- 1/2 cup strong cheddar cheese, grated and divided
- 1/4 cup parmesan cheese, grated
- 2 tablespoons butter, melted
- 1 organic egg
- 1 teaspoon fresh thyme leaves, minced

1. Preheat the oven to 350°F. Line a large baking sheet with parchment paper.
2. In a bowl, place the coconut flour, 1/4 cup of grated cheddar, parmesan, butter, and egg, and mix until well combined.
3. Make 8 equal-sized balls from the mixture.
4. Arrange the balls onto a prepared baking sheet in a single layer about 2-inch apart.
5. Form into flat discs.
6. Sprinkle each disc with the remaining cheddar, followed by thyme.
7. Bake for around 15 minutes.

Calories: 101 | Fat: 6.5g | Fiber: 1.4g | Protein: 3.1g Carbohydrates: 1.2g

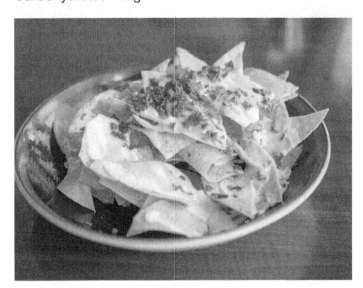

7. Bacon & Avocado Omelet

Preparation time: 5 minutes | Cooking time: 5 minutes | Servings: 1

- 1 slice crispy bacon
- 2 large organic eggs
- 5 cups freshly grated parmesan cheese
- Your choice of herbs, finely chopped
- 2 tablespoons ghee or coconut oil or butter
- Half of 1 small avocado

1. Prepare the bacon to your liking and set it aside. Combine the eggs, parmesan cheese, and your choice of finely chopped herbs. Warm a skillet and add the butter/ghee to melt using the medium-high heat setting. When the pan is hot, whisk and add the eggs.
2. Prepare the omelet working it towards the middle of the pan for about 30 seconds. When firm, flip, and cook it for another 30 seconds. Arrange the omelet on a plate and garnish with the crunched bacon bits. Serve with sliced avocado.

Carbohydrates: 3.3g | Protein: 30g | Fats: 63g
Calories: 719

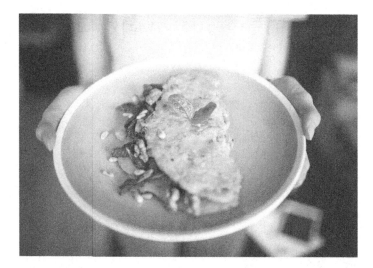

8. Basic Opie Rolls

Preparation time: 20 minutes | Cooking time: 35 minutes | Servings: 12 roll

- 1/8 teaspoon salt
- 1/8 teaspoon cream of tartar
- 3 ounces cream cheese, cubed
- 3 large eggs

1. Preheat the oven to about 300°F, then separate the egg whites from egg yolks and place both eggs in different bowls. Using an electric mixer, beat well the egg whites until the mixture is very bubbly, then add in the cream of tartar and mix again until it forms a stiff peak.
2. In the bowl, with the egg yolks, put in 3 ounces of cubed cheese and salt. Mix well until the mixture has doubled in size and is pale yellow. Put the egg white mixture into the egg yolk mixture and fold the mixture gently together.
3. Spray some oil on the cookie sheet coated with some parchment paper, then add dollops of the batter and bake for around 30 minutes.
4. You will know they are ready when the upper part of the rolls is firm and golden. Leave them to cool for a few minutes on a wire rack. Enjoy with some coffee.

Calories: 45 | Fats: 4g | Proteins: 2g
Carbohydrates: 0g

9. Bacon Hash

Preparation time: 5 minutes | Cooking time: 10 minutes | Servings: 2

- 1 small green pepper
- 2 jalapenos
- 1 small onion
- 4 eggs
- 6 bacon slices

1. Chop the bacon into chunks using a food processor. Set aside for now. Slice the onions and peppers into thin strips. Dice the jalapenos as small as possible.
2. Heat a skillet and fry the veggies. Once browned, combine the fixings and cook until crispy. Place on a serving dish with the eggs.

Carbohydrates: 9g | Protein: 23g | Fats: 24
Calories: 366

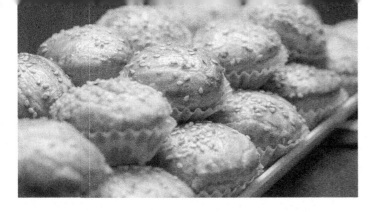

10. Bacon & Egg Breakfast Muffins

Preparation time: 15 minutes | Cooking time: 30 minutes | Servings: 12

8 large eggs
8 slices bacon
2/3 cup green onion

1. Warm the oven at 350°F. Spritz the muffin tin wells using a cooking oil spray. Chop the onions and set them aside.
2. Prepare a large skillet using the medium temperature setting. Fry the bacon until it's crispy and place it on a layer of paper towels to drain the grease. Chop it into small pieces after it has cooled.
3. Whisk the eggs, bacon, and green onions, mixing well until all of the fixings are incorporated. Dump the egg mixture into the muffin tin (halfway full). Bake it for about 20 to 25 minutes. Cool slightly and serve.

Carbohydrates: 0.4g | Protein: 5.6g | Fats: 4.9g
Calories: 69

11. Bacon & Cheese Frittata

Preparation time: 5 minutes | Cooking time: 5 minutes | Servings: 6

1 cup heavy cream
6 eggs
5 crispy slices of bacon
2 chopped green onions
4 ounces cheddar cheese
Salt and pepper

1. Warm the oven temperature to reach 350°F.
2. Whisk the eggs and seasonings. Empty into the pie pan and top off with the remainder of the fixings. Bake 30–35 minutes. Wait for a few minutes before serving for the best result.

Carbohydrates: 2g | Protein: 13g | Fats: 29g
Calories: 320

12. Baked Apples

Preparation time: 10 minutes | Cooking time: 1 hours | Servings: 4

4 teaspoons keto-friendly sweetener.
1 1/2 teaspoons cinnamon
1/4 cup chopped pecans
4 large granny smith apples

1. Set the oven temperature at 375°F. Mix the sweetener with cinnamon and pecans. Core the apple and add the prepared stuffing.
2. Add enough water into the baking dish to cover the bottom of the apple. Bake them for about 45 minutes to 1 hour.

Carbohydrates: 16g | Protein: 6.8g | Fats: 19.9g
Calories: 175

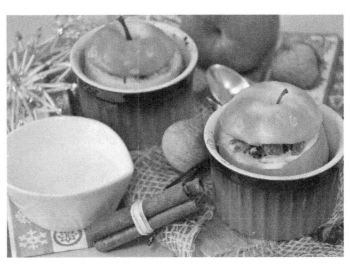

13. Parsley Soufflé

Preparation time: 5 minutes | Cooking time: 6 minutes | Servings: 1

2 eggs
1 red chili pepper
2 tablespoons coconut
cream
1 tablespoon parsley
Salt

1. Blend all the soufflé items into a food processor.
2. Put it in the soufflé dishes, then bake within 6 minutes at 390°F. Serve.

Calories: 108 | Total fat: 9g | Cholesterol: 180mg
Sodium: 146mg | Total carbs: 1.1g | Protein: 6g

14. Tofu Mushrooms

Preparation time: 5 minutes | Cooking time: 10 minutes | Servings: 3

- 1 block of tofu, cubed
- 1 cup mushrooms
- 4 tablespoons butter
- 4 tablespoons parmesan cheese
- Salt
- Ground black pepper

1. Toss the tofu cubes with melted butter, salt, and black pepper in a mixing bowl.
2. Sauté the tofu within 5 minutes. Stir in cheese and mushrooms.
3. Sauté for another 5 minutes. Serve.

Calories: 211 | Total fat: 18.5g | Cholesterol: 51mg
Sodium: 346mg | Total carbs: 2g | Protein: 11.5g

15. Onion Tofu

Preparation time: 8 minutes | Cooking time: 5 minutes | Servings: 3

- 2 blocks of tofu
- 2 onions
- 2 tablespoons butter
- 1 cup cheddar cheese
- Salt
- Ground black pepper

1. Rub the tofu with salt and pepper in a bowl.
2. Add melted butter and onions to a skillet to sauté within 3 minutes.
3. Toss in tofu and stir cook for 2 minutes. Stir in cheese and cover the skillet for 5 minutes on low heat. Serve.

Calories: 184 | Total fat: 12.7g | Total carbs: 6.3g
Sugar: 2.7g | Fiber: 1.6g | Protein: 12.2g

16. Spinach-Rich Ballet

Preparation time: 5 minutes | Cooking time: 30 minutes | Servings: 4

- 1 1/2 pounds baby spinach
- 8 teaspoons coconut cream
- 14 ounces cauliflower
- 2 tablespoons unsalted butter
- Salt
- Ground black pepper

1. Warm-up oven at 360°F.
2. Melt butter, then toss in spinach to sauté for 3 minutes.
3. Divide the spinach into 4 ramekins.
4. Divide cream, cauliflower, salt, and black pepper in the ramekins.
5. Bake within 25 minutes. Serve.

Calories: 188 | Total fat: 12.5g | Cholesterol: 53mg
Sodium: 1098mg | Total carbs: 4.9g | Protein: 14.6g

17. Nut Porridge

Preparation time: 10 minutes | Cooking time: 15 minutes | Servings: 4

- 1 cup cashew nuts
- 1 cup pecans
- 2 tablespoons stevia
- 4 teaspoons coconut oil
- 2 cups water

1. Grind the cashews and pecans in a processor.
2. Stir in stevia, oil, and water. Add the mixture to a saucepan and cook within 5 minutes on high. Adjust on low within 10 minutes. Serve.

Calories: 260 | Total fat: 22.9g | Sodium: 9mg
Total carbs: 12.7g | Sugar: 1.8g | Fiber: 1.4g
Protein: 5.6g

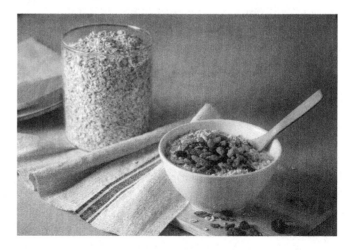

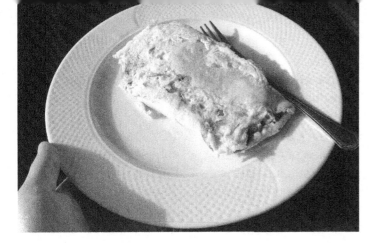

18. Pepperoni Egg Omelet

Preparation time: 5 minutes | Cooking time: 20 minutes | Servings: 4

15 pepperonis
6 eggs
2 tablespoons butter
4 tablespoons coconut cream
Salt and ground black pepper

1. Whisk eggs with pepperoni, cream, salt, and black pepper in a bowl.
2. Add 1/4 of the butter to a warm-up pan.
3. Now pour 1/4 of the batter in this melted butter and cook for 2 minutes on each side. Serve.

Calories: 141 | Total fat: 11.3g | Cholesterol: 181mg
Sodium: 334mg | Protein: 8.9g

19. Bok Choy Samba

Preparation time: 5 minutes | Cooking time: 15 minutes | Servings: 3

1 onion
4 bok choy
4 tablespoons coconut cream
Salt
Ground black pepper
1/2 cup parmesan cheese

1. Toss bok choy with salt and black pepper.
2. Add oil to a large pan and sauté onion within 5 minutes.
3. Stir in bok choy and cream. Stir for 6 minutes.
4. Toss in cheese and cover the skillet to cook on low within 3 minutes. Serve.

Calories 112 | Total fat 4.9g | Cholesterol 10mg
Sodium 355mg | Total carbs 1.9g | Protein 3g

20. Eggs and Ham

Preparation time: 25 minutes | Cooking time: 15 minutes | Servings: 4

4 eggs
10 ham slices
4 tablespoon scallions
A pinch of black pepper
A pinch of sweet paprika
1 tablespoon melted ghee

1. Grease a muffin pan with melted ghee.
2. Divide ham slices into each muffin mold to form your cups. In a bowl; mix eggs with scallions, pepper, and paprika, and whisk well.
3. Divide this mix on top of the ham, introduce your ham cups in the oven at 400 °F and bake for 15 minutes. Leave cups to cool down before dividing on plates and serving.

Calories: 250 | Fat: 10g | Fiber: 3g | Carbs: 6g
Protein: 12g

21. Bagels with Cheese

Preparation time: 10 minutes | Cooking time: 15 minutes | Servings: 6

2 1/2 cups mozzarella cheese
1 teaspoon baking powder
3 ounces cream cheese
1 1/2 cups almond flour
2 eggs

1. Shred the mozzarella and combine with the flour, baking powder, and cream cheese in a mixing container. Put into the microwave for about 1 minute. Mix well.
2. Let the mixture cool and add the eggs. Break apart into 6 sections and shape into round bagels. Note: you can also sprinkle with a seasoning of your choice or a pinch of salt if desired.
3. Bake them for approximately 12 to 15 minutes. Serve or cool and store.

Carbohydrates: 8g| Protein: 19g | Fats: 31g
Calories: 374

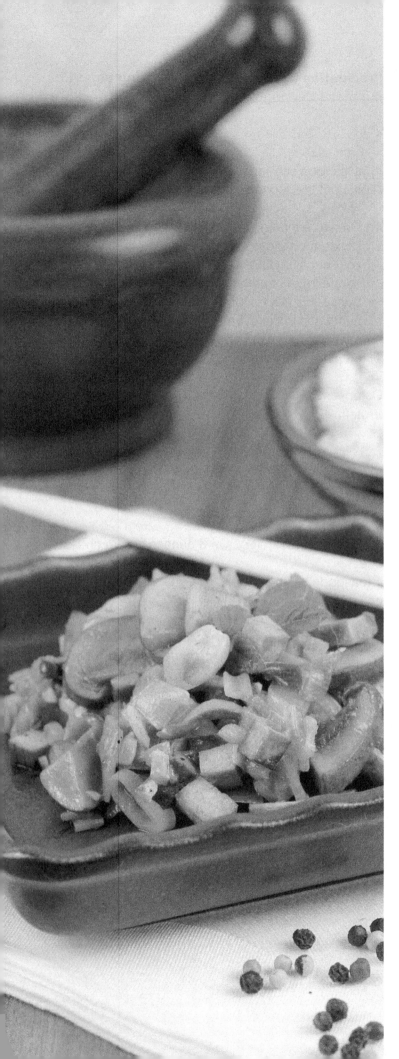

22. Breakfast Roll-Ups

Preparation time: 5 minutes | Cooking time: 15 minutes | Servings: 5 roll-ups

Non-stick cooking spray
5 patties of cooked breakfast sausage
5 slices of cooked bacon
1/2 cups cheddar cheese, shredded
Pepper and salt
10 large eggs

1. Preheat a skillet on medium to high heat, then using a whisk, combine two of the eggs in a mixing bowl.
2. After the pan has become hot, lower the heat to medium-low, then put in the eggs. If you want to, you can utilize some cooking spray.
3. Season the eggs with some pepper and salt.
4. Cover the eggs and leave them to cook for a couple of minutes or until the eggs are almost cooked.
5. Drizzle around 1/3 cup of cheese on top of the eggs, then place a strip of bacon and divide the sausage into two, and place on top.
6. Roll the egg carefully on top of the fillings. The roll-up will almost look like a taquito. If you have a hard time folding over the egg, use a spatula to keep the egg intact until the egg has molded into a roll-up.
7. Put aside the roll-up then repeat the above steps until you have 4 more roll-ups; you should have 5 roll-ups in total.

Calories: 412.2g | Fats: 31.66g | Proteins: 28.21g Carbohydrates: 2.26g

Chapter 10. Lunch Recipes

23. Slow Cooked Roasted Pork and Creamy Gravy

Preparation time: 15 minutes | Cooking time: 8 hour and 15 minutes | Servings: 6

For the creamy gravy:
2 cups whipping cream
Roast juice

For the pork:
2 pounds pork roast
1/2 tablespoon salt
3 cups water
1 bay leaf
5 black peppercorns
2 teaspoon thyme
2 garlic cloves
2 ounces ginger
1-1/3 teaspoon black pepper
1 tablespoon of each:
Paprika powder
Olive oil

1. Warm up your oven at 200°F.
2. Add the meat, salt, and water to a baking dish. Put peppercorns, thyme, and bay leaf. Put in the oven within 8 hours. Remove. Reserve the juices. Adjust to 400°F.
3. Put ginger, garlic, pepper, and oil. Rub the mixture on the meat. Roast the pork within 15 minutes.
4. Slice the roasted meat. Strain the meat juices in a bowl. Boil for reducing it by half.
5. Add the cream. Simmer within 20 minutes. Serve with creamy gravy.

Calories: 586.9 | Protein: 27.9g | Carbs: 2.6g
Fat: 50.3g | Fiber: 1.5g

24. Grilled Salmon and Zucchini with Mango Sauce

Preparation time: 5 minutes | Cooking time: 10 minutes | Servings: 4

4 (6-ounce) boneless salmon fillets
1 tablespoon olive oil
Salt and pepper
1 large zucchini, sliced in coins
2 tablespoons fresh lemon juice
1/2 cup chopped mango
1/4 cup fresh chopped cilantro
1 teaspoon lemon zest
1/2 cup canned coconut milk

1. Preheat a grill pan to heat and sprinkle with cooking spray.
2. Brush the salmon with olive oil and season with salt and pepper.
3. Apply lemon juice to the zucchini and season with salt and pepper.
4. Put the zucchini and salmon fillets on the grill pan.
5. Cook for 5 minutes then turn all over and cook for another 5 minutes.
6. Combine the remaining ingredients in a blender to create a sauce.
7. Serve the side-drizzled salmon filets with mango sauce and zucchini.

Calories: 350 | Fat: 21.5g | Protein: 35g
Carbohydrates: 8g | Sugar: 2g | Net carbs: 6g

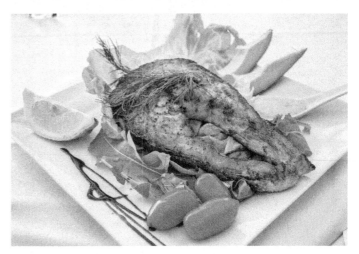

25. Crispy Cuban Pork Roast

Preparation time: 15 minutes | Cooking time: 4 minutes | Servings: 6

5 pounds pork shoulder
4 teaspoons salt
2 teaspoons cumin
1 teaspoon black pepper
2 tablespoons oregano
1 red onion
4 garlic cloves
Orange juice
2 lemons juiced
1-1/4 cup olive oil

1. Rub the pork shoulder with salt in a bowl. Mix all the remaining items in a blender to make the marinade.
2. Marinate the meat within 8 hours. Cook within 40 minutes. Warm up your oven at 400°F. Roast the pork within 30 minutes.
3. Remove the meat juice. Simmer within 20 minutes. Shred the meat.
4. Pour the meat juice. Serve.

Calories: 910.3 | Protein: 58.3g | Carbs: 5.3g
Fat: 69.6g | Fiber: 2.2g

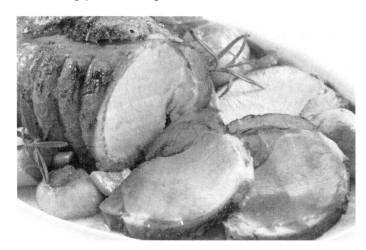

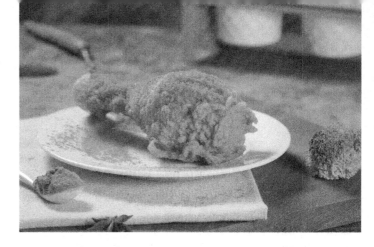

26. Garlic Chicken

Preparation time: 15 minutes | Cooking time: 40 minutes | Servings: 4

2 ounces butter
2 pounds chicken drumsticks
Pepper
Salt
Lemon juice
2 tablespoons olive oil
7 garlic cloves
1/2 cup parsley

1. Warm-up oven at 480°F.
2. Put the chicken in a greased baking dish. Add pepper and salt.
3. Add olive oil with lemon juice over the chicken. Sprinkle parsley and garlic on top.
4. Bake within 40 minutes. Serve.

Calories: 540.3 | Protein: 41.3g | Carbs: 3.1g
Fat: 38.6g | Fiber: 1.6g

27. Chicken Broccoli Lunch

Preparation time: 10 minutes | Cooking time: 5 minutes | Servings: 1

1 roasted chicken leg
1/2 cup broccoli florets
1/2 tablespoon unsalted
butter softened
2 garlic cloves, minced
Salt and pepper to taste

1. Boil the broccoli in lightly salted water for 5 minutes. Drain the water from the pot and keep the broccoli in the pot. Keep the lid on to keep the broccoli warm.
2. Mix all the butter, garlic, salt, and pepper in a small bowl to create the garlic butter.
3. Place the chicken, broccoli, and garlic butter. Serve.

Calories: 257 | Carbs: 5.1g | Fat: 14 | Protein: 27.4g

28. Keto Barbecued Ribs

Preparation time: 15 minutes | Cooking time: 1 hour 10 minutes | Servings: 4

1-1/4 cup Dijon mustard	1 1/2 tablespoons garlic powder
3 pounds spare ribs	2 1/2 tablespoon black pepper
4 tablespoons paprika powder	
1/2 tablespoon chili powder	

2 teaspoons of each:
Onion powder   Cumin

2 tablespoons of each:
Cider vinegar   Salt
Butter

1. Warm up a grill for 30 minutes.
2. Mix vinegar and Dijon mustard in a bowl; put the ribs and coat.
3. Mix all the listed spices. Rub the mix all over the ribs. Put aside. Put ribs on an aluminum foil. Add some butter over the ribs. Wrap with foil. Grill within 1 hour. Remove and slice.
4. Put the reserved spice mix. Grill again within 10 minutes. Serve.

Calories: 980.3 | Protein: 54.3g | Carbs: 5.8g
Fat: 80.2g | Fiber: 4.6g

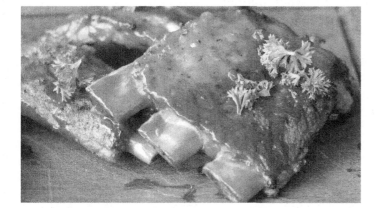

29. Chicken Wings and Blue Cheese Dressing

Preparation time: 70 minutes | Cooking time: 25 minutes | Servings: 4

For the blue cheese dressing:

1-1/3 cup mayonnaise	3 ounces blue cheese
1-1/4 cup sour cream	1-1/4 teaspoon of each:
3 teaspoons lemon juice	Salt
1/2 cup whipping cream	Garlic powder

For the chicken wings:

2 pounds chicken wings	1-1/3 teaspoon black pepper
2 tablespoons olive oil	1 teaspoon salt
1-1/4 teaspoon garlic powder	2 ounces parmesan cheese
1 garlic clove	

1. Mix all the blue cheese dressing items in a bowl. Chill within 40 minutes.
2. Combine the chicken with olive oil and spices. Marinate for 30 minutes.
3. Bake in the oven for 25 minutes. Toss the chicken wings with parmesan cheese in a bowl.
4. Serve with blue cheese dressing by the side.

Calories: 839.3 | Protein: 51.2g | Carbs: 2.9g
Fat: 67.8g | Fiber: 0.2g

30. Cheesy Chicken Cauliflower

Preparation time: 5 minutes | Cooking time: 10 minutes | Servings: 4

2 cups cauliflower florets, chopped	1/4 cup shredded cheddar cheese
1/2 cup red bell pepper, chopped	1 tablespoon sour cream
1 tablespoon butter	Salt and pepper to taste
1 cup roasted chicken, shredded	

1. Stir fry the cauliflower and peppers in the butter over medium heat until the veggies are tender.
2. Add the chicken and cook until the chicken is warmed through.
3. Add the remaining ingredients: and stir until the cheese is melted.
4. Serve warm.

Calories: 144 | Carbs: 4g | Fat: 8.5g | Protein: 13.2 g.

31. Keto Hamburger

Preparation time: 15 minutes | Cooking time: 70 minutes | Servings: 4

For the burger buns:
- 2 cups almond flour
- 5 tablespoons ground psyllium husk powder
- 2 teaspoons baking powder
- 1 teaspoon salt
- 1 + 1/2 cup water
- 2 teaspoons cider vinegar
- 3 egg whites
- 1 tablespoon sesame seed

For the hamburger:
- 2 pounds beef
- 1-ounce olive oil
- Pepper and salt
- 1 1/2-ounce lettuce
- 1 tomato
- 1 red onion
- 1/2 cup mayonnaise
- 5 ounces bacon

1. Warm up your oven at 300°F.
2. Mix the listed dry items for the buns in a bowl. Boil the water. Put egg whites, water, and vinegar into the dry mix. Mix.
3. Make individual pieces of buns, put sesame seeds on the top. Bake for 60 minutes
4. Fry the slices of bacon. Keep aside.
5. Mix beef, pepper, and salt in a bowl. Make patties. Grill the beef patties for 5 minutes, each side.
6. Combine mayonnaise and lettuce in a bowl. Cut the buns in half. Add beef patty, lettuce mix, onion slice, and a tomato slice. Top with bacon slices. Serve.

Calories: 1070.3 | Protein: 53.4g | Carbs: 6.1g
Fat: 85.3g | Fiber: 12.3g

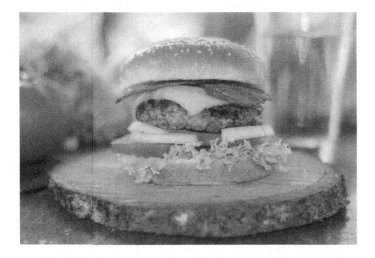

32. Turkey and Cream Cheese Sauce

Preparation time: 15 minutes | Cooking time: 25 minutes | Servings: 5

- 2 tablespoons butter
- 2 pounds turkey breast
- 2 cups whipping cream
- 7 ounces cream cheese
- 1 tablespoon tamari soy sauce
- Pepper
- Salt
- 1- + 1/2-ounces capers

1. Warm up the oven at 340°F, then dissolves half the butter in an iron skillet.
2. Rub the turkey breast with pepper and salt. Fry within 5 minutes.
3. Bake within 10 minutes.
4. Add the drippings of turkey in a pan, cream cheese, and whipping cream. Simmer. Add pepper, soy sauce, and salt.
5. Sauté the small capers in the remaining butter.
6. Slice and serve with fried capers and cream cheese sauce.

Calories: 810.3 | Protein: 47.6g | Carbs: 6.9g
Fat: 68.6g | Fiber: 0.6g

33. Baked Salmon and Pesto

Preparation time: 15 minutes | Cooking time: 30 minutes | Servings: 4

For the green sauce:
- 4 tablespoons green pesto
- 1 cup mayonnaise
- 1/2 cup Greek yogurt
- Pepper
- Salt

For the salmon:
- 2 pounds salmon
- 4 tablespoons green pesto
- Pepper
- Salt

1. Put the fillets on a greased baking dish with the skin side down. Add pesto on top. Add pepper and salt.
2. Bake at 400°F within 30 minutes.
3. Combine all the listed fixing for the green sauce in a bowl.
4. Serve the baked salmon with green sauce on top.

Calories: 1010.2 | Protein: 51.6g | Carbs: 3.1g
Fat: 87.6g | Fiber: 0.7g

34. Salmon Burgers with Lemon Butter and Mash

Preparation time: 70 minutes | Cooking time: 15 minutes | Servings: 4

For the salmon burgers:
- 2 pounds salmon
- 1 egg
- 1/2 yellow onion
- 1 teaspoon salt
- 1/2 teaspoon black pepper
- 2 ounces butter

For the green mash:
- 1-pound broccoli
- 5 ounces butter
- 2 ounces parmesan cheese
- Pepper
- Salt

For the lemon butter:
- 4 ounces butter
- 2 tablespoons lemon juice
- Pepper
- Salt

1. Warm up your oven at 200°F.
2. Cut the salmon into small pieces. Combine all the burger items with the fish in a blender. Pulse for 30 seconds. Make 8 patties.
3. Warm-up butter in an iron skillet. Fry the burgers for 5 minutes.
4. Boil water, along with some salt in a pot, put the broccoli florets. Cook for 3 to 4 minutes. Drain. Add parmesan cheese and butter. Blend the ingredients using an immersion blender. Add pepper and salt.
5. Combine lemon juice with butter, pepper, and salt. Beat using an electric beater.
6. Put a dollop of lemon butter on the top and green mash by the side. Serve.

Calories: 1025.3 | Protein: 44.5g | Carbs: 6.8g
Fat: 90.1g | Fiber: 3.1g

35. Chicken Soup

Preparation time: 10 minutes | Cooking time: 25 minutes | Servings: 6

- 2 celery stalks, chopped
- 1 cup mushrooms, sliced
- 2 garlic cloves, minced
- 2 tablespoons butter
- 6 cups chicken broth
- 1 carrot, sliced
- 1 tablespoon garlic powder
- 1 tablespoon onion powder
- Salt and pepper to taste
- 4 cups roasted chicken, shredded
- 4 cups green cabbage, sliced into strips

1. Sauté the celery, mushrooms, and garlic in the butter in a pot over medium heat for 4 minutes.
2. Add broth, carrots, garlic powder, onion powder, salt, and pepper.
3. Simmer for 10 minutes or until the vegetables are tender.
4. Add the chicken and cabbage and simmer for another 10 minutes or until the cabbage is tender.
5. Serve warm.
6. It can be refrigerated for up to 3 days or frozen for up to 1 month.

Calories: 279 | Carbs: 7.5g | Fat: 12.3g
Protein: 33.4g

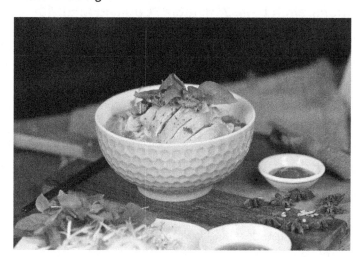

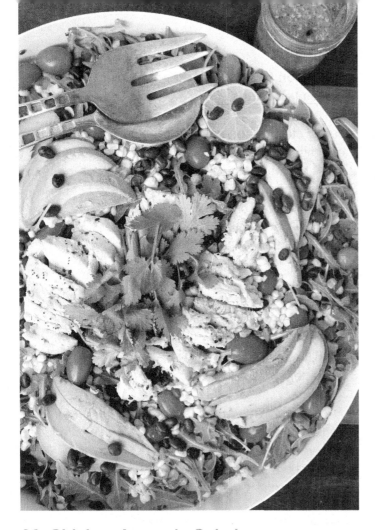

36. Chicken Avocado Salad

Preparation time: 7 minutes | Cooking time: 10 minutes | Servings: 4

1 cup roasted chicken, shredded
1 bacon strip, cooked and chopped
1/2 medium avocado, chopped
1/4 cup cheddar cheese, grated
1 hard-boiled egg, chopped
1 cup Romaine lettuce, chopped
1 tablespoon olive oil
1 tablespoon apple cider vinegar
Salt and pepper to taste

1. Create the dressing by mixing apple cider vinegar, oil, salt, and pepper.
2. Combine all the other ingredients: in a mixing bowl.
3. Drizzle with the dressing and toss. Serve.
4. It can be refrigerated for up to 3 days.

Calories: 220 | Carbs: 2.8g | Fat: 16.7g | Protein: 14.8g

37. Turkey Burgers and Tomato Butter

Preparation time: 15 minutes | Cooking time: 15 minutes | Servings: 4

For the chicken patties:
2 pounds chicken
1 egg
1/2 onion
1 teaspoon salt
1/2 teaspoon black pepper
1 1/2 teaspoon thyme
2 ounces butter

For the fried cabbage:
2 pounds green cabbage
3 ounces butter
1 teaspoon salt
1/2 teaspoon black pepper (ground)

For the tomato butter:
4 ounces butter
1 tablespoon tomato paste
1 teaspoon red wine vinegar
Pepper
Salt

1. Warm up your oven at 200°F.
2. Combine the listed items for the patties in a large bowl. Shape the mixture into patties.
3. Fry the chicken patties for 5 minutes, each side. Keep warm in the oven.
4. Warm up butter in a pan. Put the cabbage, plus pepper and salt. Fry for 5 minutes.
5. Whip the items for the tomato butter in a bowl using an electric mixer.
6. Serve with a dollop of tomato butter from the top.

Calories: 830.4 | Protein: 33.6g | Carbs: 6.7g
Fat: 71.5g | Fiber: 5.1g

38. Chicken Casserole

Preparation time: 10 minutes | Cooking time: 40 minutes | Servings: 8

- 1 pound boneless chicken breasts, cut into 1-inch cubes
- 2 tablespoons butter
- 4 tablespoons green pesto
- 1 cup heavy whipping cream
- 1/4 cup green bell peppers, diced
- 1 cup feta cheese, diced
- 1 garlic clove, minced
- Salt and pepper to taste

1. Preheat your oven to 400°F.
2. Season the chicken with salt and pepper, then batch fry in the butter until golden brown.
3. Place the fried chicken pieces in a baking dish. Add the feta cheese, garlic, and bell peppers.
4. Combine the pesto and heavy cream in a bowl. Pour on top of the chicken mixture and spread with a spatula.
5. Bake for 30 minutes or until the casserole is light brown around the edges.
6. Serve warm.
7. It can be refrigerated for up to 5 days and frozen for 2 weeks.

Calories: 294 | Carbs: 1.7g | Fat: 22.7g | Protein: 20.1g

39. Keto Chicken with Butter and Lemon

Preparation time: 15 minutes | Cooking time: 1 hours 30 minutes | Servings: 2

- 3 pounds whole chicken
- Pepper and salt
- 2 teaspoon barbecue seasoning
- 5 ounces butter
- 1 lemon
- 2 onions

1. Warm-up oven at 340°F. Grease the baking dish.
2. Rub the chicken with pepper, salt, and barbecue seasoning. Put in the baking dish.
3. Arrange lemon wedges, slices of butter, and onions surrounding the chicken.
4. Bake within 1 hour and 30 minutes. Slice and serve.

Calories: 980.3 | Protein: 57.2g | Carbs: 0.4g Fat: 81.3g | Fiber: 0.1g

40. Easy Meatballs

Preparation time: 10 minutes | Cooking time: 20 minutes | Servings: 4

- 1 pound ground beef
- 1 egg, beaten
- 2 tablespoons butter
- Salt and pepper to taste
- 1 teaspoon garlic powder
- 1 teaspoon onion powder
- 1/4 cup mayonnaise
- 1/4 cup pickled jalapeños
- 1 cup cheddar cheese, grated

1. Combine the cheese, mayonnaise, pickled jalapenos, salt, pepper, garlic powder, and onion powder in a large mixing bowl.
2. Add the beef and egg and combine using clean hands.
3. Form large meatballs. Makes about 12.
4. Fry the meatballs in the butter over medium heat for about 4 minutes on each side or until golden brown.
5. Serve warm with a keto-friendly side.
6. The meatball mixture can also be used to make a meatloaf. Just preheat your oven to 400°F, press the mixture into a loaf pan, and bake for about 30 minutes or until the top is golden brown.
7. It can be refrigerated for up to 5 days or frozen for up to 3 months.

Calories: 454 | Carbs: 5g | Fat: 28.2g | Protein: 43.2g

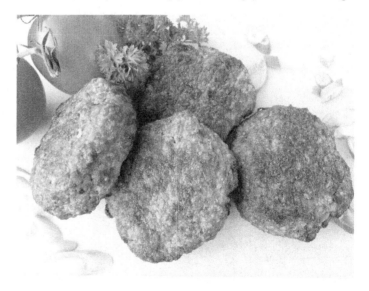

41. Buffalo Drumsticks and Chili Aioli

Preparation time: 15 minutes | Cooking time: 40 minutes | Servings: 4

2 pounds chicken drumsticks

For the chili aioli:
1/2 cup mayonnaise
1 tablespoon smoked paprika powder
1 garlic clove

For the marinade:
1 tablespoon tomato paste

2 tablespoons of each:
White wine vinegar
Olive oil

1 teaspoon of each:
Salt
Paprika powder
Tabasco

1. Warm-up oven at 400°F.
2. Combine the listed marinade fixing. Marinate the chicken drumsticks within 10 minutes.
3. Arrange the chicken drumsticks in the tray. Bake within 40 minutes.
4. Combine the listed items for the chili aioli in a bowl. Serve.

Calories: 567.8 | Protein: 41.3g | Carbs: 2.2g Fat: 43.2g | Fiber: 1.1g

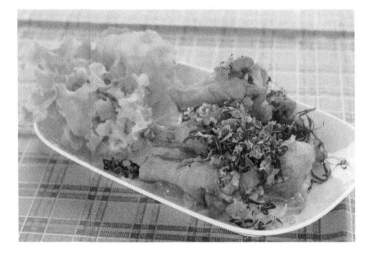

42. Italian Style Eggs

Preparation time: 25 minutes | Cooking time: 10 minutes | Servings: 1

2 eggs
1/4 teaspoon rosemary, dried
1/2 cup cherry tomatoes halved
1 1/2 cups kale, chopped
1/2 teaspoon coconut oil
3 tablespoons water
1 teaspoon balsamic vinegar
1/4 avocado, peeled and chopped

1. Heat up a pan with the oil over medium-high heat, add water, kale, rosemary, and tomatoes, stir; cover, and cook for 4 minutes.
2. Uncover the pan, stir again, and add eggs.
3. Stir and scramble eggs for 3 minutes.
4. Add vinegar, stir everything and transfer to a serving plate. Top with chopped avocado and serve.

Calories: 185 | Fat: 10g | Fiber: 1g | Carbs: 6g Protein: 7g

43. Orange and Dates Granola

Preparation time: 25 minutes | Cooking time: 6 minutes | Servings: 15

5 ounces dates, soaked in hot water
1/2 cup pumpkin seeds
Juice from 1 orange
Grated rind of 1/2 orange
1 cup desiccated coconut
1/2 cup slivered almonds
1/2 cup linseeds
1/2 cup sesame seeds
Almond milk for serving

1. In a bowl, mix almonds with orange rind, orange juice, linseeds, and coconut, pumpkin, and sesame seeds, and stir well.
2. Drain dates, add them to your food processor and blend well. Add this paste to the almonds mix and stir well again.
3. Spread this on a lined baking sheet, introduce it in the oven at 350°F and bake for 15 minutes, stirring every 4 minutes.
4. Take granola out of the oven, leave aside to cool down a bit and then serve with almond milk.

Calories: 208g | Protein: 6g | Fiber: 5 | Fat: 9 Sugar: 0

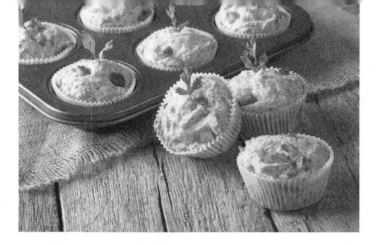

44. Bacon Muffins

Preparation time: 40 minutes | Cooking time: 4 minutes | Servings: 20

4 ounces bacon slices
3 garlic cloves, minced
1 small yellow onion, chopped
1 zucchini, thinly sliced
A handful of spinach, torn
6 canned and pickled artichoke hearts, chopped
8 eggs
1/4 teaspoon paprika
A pinch of black pepper
A pinch of cayenne pepper
1/4 cup coconut cream

1. Heat up a pan over medium-high heat, add bacon, and stir. Cook until it's crispy, transfer to paper towels, drain grease, and leave aside for now.
2. Heat up the same pan over medium heat again, add garlic and onion, stir and cook for 4 minutes.
3. In a bowl; mix eggs with coconut cream, onions, garlic, paprika, black pepper, and cayenne, and whisk well.
4. Add spinach, zucchini, and artichoke pieces and stir everything.
5. Divide crispy bacon slices in a muffin pan, add the egg mixture on top, introduce your muffins in the oven, and bake at 400°F for 20 minutes. Leave them to cool down before serving them for breakfast.

Calories: 270 | Fat: 12g | Fiber: 4g | Carbs: 6g
Protein: 12g

45. Pot Roast with Green Beans

Preparation time: 10 minutes | Cooking time: 5 hours | Servings: 8

2 medium stalks celery, sliced
1 medium yellow onion, chopped
1 (3-pound) boneless beef chuck roast
Salt and pepper
1/4 cup beef broth
2 tablespoons Worcestershire sauce
4 cups green beans, trimmed
2 tablespoons cold butter, chopped

1. In a pot, add celery and onion.
2. Put the beef on top and season with salt and pepper.
3. Whisk the beef broth and Worcestershire sauce together, then pour in.
4. Cover and cook for 5 hours on low heat, until the beef is very tender.
5. Bring the beef off on a cutting board and cut it into chunks.
6. Return the beef to the pot and add the chopped butter and the beans.
7. Cover and cook for 20 to 30 minutes on warm, until the beans are tender.

Calories: 375 | Fat: 13.5g | Protein: 53g
Carbohydrates: 6g | Fiber: 2g | Net carbs: 4g

46. Salmon Skewers Wrapped with Prosciutto

Preparation time: 15 minutes | Cooking time: 4 minutes | Servings: 4

1/4 cup basil
1-pound salmon
1 pinch of black pepper
4 ounces prosciutto
1 tablespoon olive oil
8 skewers

1. Start by soaking the skewers in a bowl of water.
2. Cut the salmon fillets lengthwise. Thread the salmon using skewers.
3. Coat the skewers in pepper and basil. Wrap the slices of prosciutto around the salmon.
4. Warm up oil in a grill pan. Grill the skewers within 4 minutes. Serve.

Calories: 670.5 | Protein: 27.2g | Carbs: 1.2g
Fat: 61.6g | Fiber: 0.3g

Chapter 11 Snacks

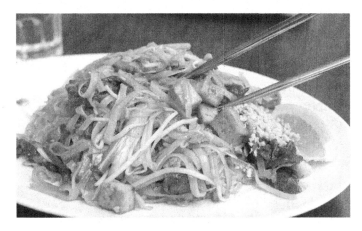

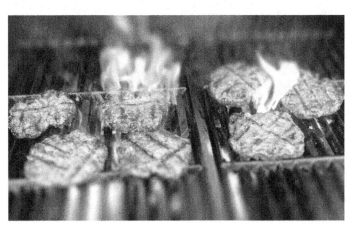

47. Baked Zucchini Noodles with Feta

Preparation time: 15 minutes | Cooking time: 15 minutes | Servings: 1

1 quartered plum tomato
2 spiralized zucchini
8 cubes feta cheese
1 teaspoon pepper
Salt
1 tablespoon olive oil
3 tablespoons olive oil

1. Set the oven temperature to reach 375°F.
2. Slice the zucchini noodles with a spiralizer and put the olive oil, tomato, pepper, and salt.
3. Bake within 10 to 15 minutes. Transfer, then put cheese cubes; toss. Serve.

Carbohydrates: 5g | Protein: 4g | Total Fats: 8g
Calories: 105

48. Brussels Sprouts with Bacon

Preparation time: 15 minutes | Cooking time: 40 minutes | Servings: 6

16 ounces bacon
Black pepper
16 ounces Brussels sprouts

1. Warm the oven to reach 400°F.
2. Slice the bacon into small lengthwise pieces. Put the sprouts and bacon with pepper.
3. Bake within 35 to 40 minutes. Serve.

Carbohydrates: 3.9g | Protein: 7.9g | Total Fats: 6.9g
Calories: 113

49. Bunless Burger—Keto Style

Preparation time: 15 minutes | Cooking time: 25 minutes | Servings: 6

1 pound ground beef
1 tablespoon Worcestershire sauce
1 tablespoon steak seasoning
2 tablespoons olive oil
4 ounces onions

1. Mix the beef, olive oil, Worcestershire sauce, and seasonings.
2. Grill the burger. Prepare onions by adding 1 tablespoon of oil in a skillet to med-low heat.

Carbohydrates: 2g | Protein: 26g | Total Fats: 40g
Calories: 479

50. Coffee BBQ Pork Belly

Preparation time: 15 minutes | Cooking time: 60 minutes | Servings: 4

1.5 cups beef stock
2 pounds pork belly
4 tablespoons olive oil
Low-carb barbecue dry rub
2 tablespoons instant espresso powder

1. Set the oven at 350°F.
2. Heat up the beef stock in a small saucepan.
3. Mix in the dry barbecue rub and espresso powder.
4. Put the pork belly, skin side up in a shallow dish and drizzle half of the oil over the top.
5. Put hot stock around the pork belly. Bake 45 min.
6. Sear each slice within 3 minutes per side. Serve.

Carbohydrates: 3.9g | Protein: 7.9g | Total Fats: 6.9g
Calories: 113

51. Salsa Turkey Cutlet and Zucchini Stir-Fry

Preparation time: 10 minutes | Cooking time: 15 minutes | Servings: 4

2 tablespoons olive oil
1 pound (454 grams) turkey cutlets
1 red onion, sliced
2 garlic cloves, minced
1 chili pepper, chopped
Sea salt and ground black pepper, to taste
1/2 teaspoon cayenne pepper
1/2 teaspoon dried basil
1 teaspoon dried rosemary
1/2 teaspoon cumin seeds
1/2 teaspoon mustard seeds
1 zucchini, spiralized
1/2 cup salsa

1. Heat 1 tablespoon of the olive oil in a frying pan over a moderate flame. Cook the turkey cutlets until they are golden brown or for about 10 minutes; shred the meat with two forks and reserve.
2. Heat the remaining tablespoon of olive oil in the same frying pan. Now, sauté the onion, garlic, and chili pepper until they have softened.
3. Add the spices and stir in the reserved turkey. Fold in the zucchini and cook for 3 minutes or until it is tender and everything is cooked through. Serve with salsa on the side. Enjoy!

Calories: 211 | Fat: 9.1g | Protein: 26.1g
Carbs: 5.5g | Net carbs: 4.4g | Fiber: 1.1g

52. Ranch Turkey with Greek Aioli Sauce

Preparation time: 10 minutes | Cooking time: 15 minutes | Servings: 4

2 eggs
Kosher salt and ground black pepper, to taste
1 teaspoon paprika
2 tablespoons pork rinds
2 tbs flaxseed meal
1/2 cup almond meal
1 pound turkey tenders, 1/2-inch thick
2 tbs sesame seeds
2 tablespoons olive oil

Sauce
2 tablespoons Greek aioli
1/2 cup Greek yogurt
Flaky sea salt and freshly ground black pepper, to season

1. Brush a baking pan with 1 tablespoon of olive oil. Bruch the chicken cutlets with the remaining tablespoon of olive oil.
2. Season the chicken cutlets with cayenne pepper, oregano, salt, and black pepper. Spread mustard on one side of each chicken cutlet.
3. Divide the garlic, peppers, and Romano cheese on the mustard side. Roll up tightly and use toothpicks to secure your rolls. Transfer to the prepared baking pan.
4. Bake in the preheated oven at 370°F for about 30 minutes until golden brown on all sides (an instant-read thermometer should register 165°F).
5. Spoon the sauerkraut over the chicken and serve.

Calories: 530 | Fat: 39g | Protein: 33g
Carbs: 6.7g | Net carbs: 5g | Fiber: 1.7g

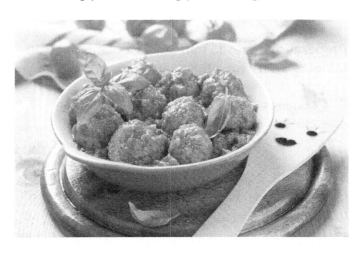

53. Fried Turkey and Pork Meatballs

Preparation time: 20minutes | Cooking time: 15 minutes | Servings: 4

4 spring onions, finely chopped
2 spring garlic stalks, chopped
2 tablespoons cilantro, chopped
1/2 pound (227 grams) ground pork
1/2 pound (227 grams) ground turkey
1 egg, whisked
1/2 cup Parmesan cheese, grated
1 teaspoon dried rosemary
1/2 teaspoon mustard powder
Sea salt and freshly ground black pepper, to season
2 tablespoons olive oil

1. In a mixing bowl, thoroughly combine all ingredients, except the olive oil. Shape small balls. Refrigerate your meatballs for 1 hour.
2. Then, heat the olive oil in a frying pan over
3. medium-high heat. Once hot, fry the meatballs for 6 minutes until nicely browned.
4. Turn them and cook for 6 minutes on other side.

Calories: 367 | Fat: 27.6g | Protein: 26g
Carbs: 3g | Net carbs: 2.5g | Fiber: 0.5g

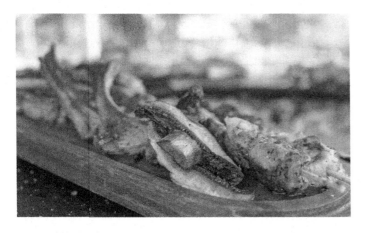

54. Garlic & Thyme Lamb Chops

Preparation time: 15 minutes | Cooking time: 10 minutes | Servings: 6

6–4 ounces lamb chops
4 whole garlic cloves
2 thyme sprigs
1 teaspoon ground thyme
3 tablespoons olive oil

1. Warm up a skillet. Put the olive oil. Rub the chops with the spices.
2. Put the chops in the skillet with the garlic and sprigs of thyme. Sauté within 3-4 mins and serve.

Calories: 252 | Fat: 21g | Net Carbohydrates: 1g
Sugar: 4g | Protein: 14g

55. Whole Chicken with Leek and Mushrooms

Preparation time: 15 minutes | Cooking time: 45 minutes | Servings: 4

1 tbs olive oil
1 1/2 pounds (680 grams) whole chicken, skinless and boneless
2 cups button mushrooms, sliced
1 serrano pepper, sliced
1 medium leek, chopped
1 teaspoon ginger-garlic paste
1/4 cup dry red wine
Sea salt, ground black pepper, to season
2 tablespoons capers
1 cup tomato paste

1. Heat the olive oil in frying pan on moderate flame. Fry the chicken until golden brown on all sides or about 10 minutes; set aside.
2. Cook mushrooms, serrano pepper, and leek in the pan drippings. Cook until softened in 6 mins.
3. Stir the ginger-garlic paste and fry for 30 secs. Add a splash of red wine to deglaze the pan.
4. Add chicken to the frying pan. Add in salt, black pepper, capers, and tomato paste; stir to combine well and bring to a rapid boil.
5. Turn the heat to medium-low and let it cook for 30 mins until everything is heated through.

Calories: 425 | Fat: 29.1g | Protein: 33.4g
Carbs: 5.6g | Net carbs: 4.4g | Fiber: 1.2g

56. Mixed Vegetable Patties

Preparation time: 15 minutes | Cooking time: 10 minutes | Servings: 4

1 cup cauliflower florets
1 bag vegetables
1.5 cups water
1 cup flax meal
2 tablespoons olive oil

1. Steam the veggies to steamer basket in 4-5 mins.
2. Mash in the flax meal. Shape into 4 patties.
3. Cook the patties within 3 minutes per side. Serve.

Net Carbohydrates: 3g | Protein: 4g
Total Fats: 10g | Calories: 220

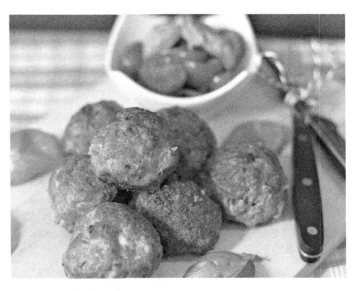

57. Keto Meatballs

Preparation time: 15 minutes | Cooking time: 20 minutes | Servings: 10

1 egg
1/2 cup grated parmesan
1/2 cup shred mozzarella
1 pound ground beef
1 tablespoon garlic

1. Warm up the oven to reach 400°F. Combine all of the fixings. Shape into meatballs. Bake within 18–20 minutes. Cool and serve.

Net Carbohydrates: 0.7g | Protein: 12.2g
Total Fats: 10.9g | Calories: 153

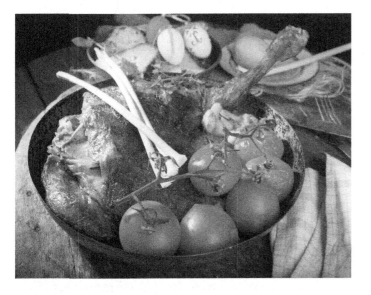

58. Roasted Leg of Lamb

Preparation time: 15 minutes | Cooking time: 1hour 30 minutes | Servings: 6

1/2 cup reduced-sodium beef broth
2-pound lamb leg
6 garlic cloves
1 tablespoon rosemary leaves
1 teaspoon black pepper

1. Warm-up oven temperature to 400°F.
2. Put the lamb in the pan and the broth and seasonings.
3. Roast for 30 minutes and lower the heat to 350°F. Cook within 1 hour.
4. Cool and serve.

Net Carbohydrates: 1g | Protein: 22g
Total Fats: 14g | Calories: 223

59. Skillet Fried Cod

Preparation time: 15 minutes | Cooking time: 30 minutes Servings: 4

6 garlic cloves
3 tablespoon ghee
4 cod fillets
Pepper and salt
Optional: Garlic powder

1. Toss half of the garlic into a skillet with the ghee.
2. Put the fillets in the pan, put garlic, pepper, salt.
3. Turn it over, and add the remainder of the minced garlic. Cook.

Net Carbohydrates: 3g | Protein: 21g
Total Fats: 42g | Calories: 470

60. Steak Pinwheels

Preparation time: 15 minutes | Cooking time: 25 minutes | Servings: 6

2-pound flank steak
1 bunch of spinach
8-ounce package mozzarella cheese

1. Warm up the oven to reach 350°F.
2. Slice steak into 6 portions. Beat thin with a mallet.
3. Shred the cheese using a food processor, sprinkle the steak. Roll it up and tie it with cooking twine.
4. Line the pan with the pinwheels and place it on a layer of spinach. Bake within 25 minutes.

Net Carbohydrates: 2g | Protein: 55g
Total Fats: 20g | Calories: 414

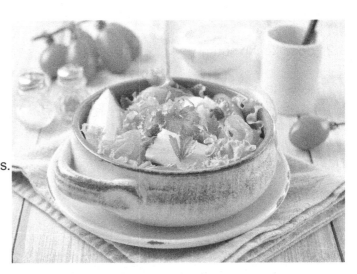

61. Salmon Pasta

Preparation time: 15 minutes | Cooking time: 1hour 30 minutes Servings: 2

2 tbss coconut oil
2 zucchinis
8 ounce smoked salmon
1/4 cup keto-friendly mayo

1. Make noodle-like strands from the zucchini.
2. Warm up the oil, put the salmon, sauté 2-3 mins.
3. Stir in the noodles and sauté for 1-2 more mins.
4. Stir in the mayo and serve.

Net Carbohydrates: 3g | Protein: 21g
Total Fats: 42g | Calories: 470

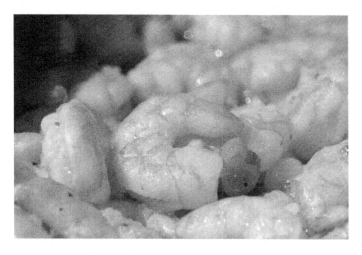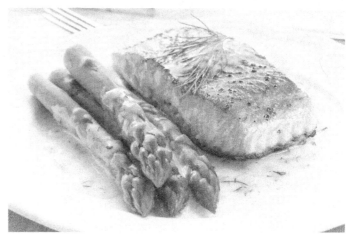

62. Tangy Shrimp

Preparation time: 15 minutes | Cooking time: 15 minutes | Servings: 2

3 garlic
1/4 cup olive oil
1/2 pound jumbo shrimp
1 lemon
Cayenne pepper, to taste

1. Sauté the garlic and cayenne with olive oil. Peel and devein the shrimp. Put pepper, salt, lemon wedges. Use the garlic oil for dipping sauce.

Net Carbohydrates: 3g | Protein: 23g
Total Fats: 27g | Calories: 335

63. Chicken Thighs with Caesar Salad

Preparation time: 15 minutes | Cooking time: 15 minutes | Servings: 4

Chicken
4 chicken thighs
1/4 cup lemon juice
2 garlic cloves, minced
2 tablespoons olive oil
2 tablespoons olive oil

Salad
1/2 cup Caesar salad dressing
12 bok choy leaves
3 parmesan cheese crisp
Parmesan cheese, grated

1. Combine the chicken ingredients in a Ziploc bag. Seal the bag, shake and refrigerate 1 hour. Preheat the grill to medium heat, and grill the chicken for about 4 minutes per side.
2. Cut bok choy leaves lengthwise, and brush them with oil. Grill 3 minutes. Place on a serving platter. Top with the chicken, and drizzle the dressing over. Sprinkle with Parmesan cheese and finish with Parmesan crisps to serve.

Calories: 530 | Fat: 39g | Protein: 33g
Carbs: 6.7g | Net carbs: 5g | Fiber: 1.7g

64. Grilled Pesto Salmon with Asparagus

Preparation time: 5 minutes | Cooking time: 15 minutes | Servings: 4

4 (6-ounce) boneless salmon fillets
1 bunch asparagus, ends trimmed
2 tablespoons olive oil
1/4 cup basil pesto
Cayenne pepper, to taste
Salt and pepper

1. Preheat the grill to heat, and oil the grills.
2. Season the salmon with salt and pepper and sprinkle with spray to cook.
3. Grill the salmon on each side for 4 to 5 minutes, until cooked.
4. Throw the asparagus with oil and grill for about 10 minutes, until tender.
5. Spoon the salmon with the pesto, and serve with the asparagus.

Calories 300 | Fat 17.5g | Protein 34.5g
Carbohydrates 2.5g | Fiber 1.5g | Net carbs 1g

65. Jamaican Jerk Pork Roast

Preparation time: 15 minutes | Cooking time: 4 hours | Servings: 12

1 tablespoon olive oil
4 pounds pork shoulder
1/2 cup beef broth
1/4 cup Jamaican Jerk spice blend

1. Rub the pork well with the oil and the jerk spice blend. Sear the roast on all sides. Put beef broth.
2. Simmer within 4 hours on low. Shred and serve.

Net Carbohydrates: 0g | Protein: 23g | Total Fats: 20g
Calories: 282

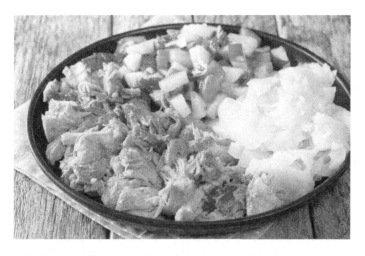

66. Slow-Cooked Kalua Pork & Cabbage

Preparation time: 15 minutes | Cooking time: 11 hours | Servings: 12

3-pound pork shoulder
1 medium cabbage
7 strips bacon
1 tbs coarse sea salt

1. Trim the fat from the roast.
2. Layer most of the bacon in the cooker. Put salt over the roast and add to the pot on top of the bacon. Cook on low within 8 to 10 hours. Put in the cabbage, and cook within an hour.
3. Shred the roast. Serve with cabbage & meat juice.

Net Carbohydrates: 4g | Protein: 22g
Total Fats: 13g | Calories: 227

67. Chicken Wing and Italian Pepper Soup

Preparation time: 15 minutes | Cooking time: 50 minutes | Servings: 6

1 tablespoon olive oil
2 pound chicken wings
1 Italian pepper, deveined and sliced
1/2 cup celery, chopped
1/2 cup onions, finely chopped
2 rosemary sprigs, leaves picked
2 thyme sprigs, leaves picked
Sea salt and ground black pepper, to taste
2 cups vegetable stock
1 whole egg

1. Heat the olive oil in a soup pot over a moderate flame. Brown the chicken wings for 4 to 5 minutes per side or until no longer pink; reserve.
2. Then, cook the Italian pepper, celery, and onions in the same pot until they have softened.
3. Stir in the rosemary, thyme, salt, black pepper, and vegetable stock; return the chicken to the pot.
4. Stir with a spoon and bring to a boil. Reduce the heat to medium-low and let it simmer an additional 45 minutes, stirring once or twice.
5. Transfer the chicken to a cutting board and shred the chicken, discarding the bones.
6. Add the egg to the pot and whisk until well combined. Add the chicken back to the pot, stir, and serve warm. Enjoy!

Calories: 284 | Fat: 18.8g | Protein: 25.3g
Carbs: 2.5g | Net carbs: 2.1g | Fiber: 0.4g

68. Pepper, Cheese, Sauerkraut Stuffed Chicken

Preparation time: 15 minutes | Cooking time: 30 minutes | Servings: 5

1 pound chicken cutlets
1/2 teaspoon cayenne pepper
1/2 teaspoon oregano
Sea salt and ground black pepper, to taste
2 garlic cloves, minced
5 Italian peppers, deveined and chopped
2 tablespoons olive oil
1 chili pepper, chopped
1 cup Romano cheese, shredded
5 tablespoons sauerkraut, for serving
1 tablespoon Dijon mustard

1. Brush a baking pan with 1 tablespoon of olive oil. Bruch the chicken cutlets with the remaining tablespoon of olive oil.
2. Season the chicken cutlets with cayenne pepper, oregano, salt, and black pepper. Spread mustard on one side of each chicken cutlet.
3. Divide the garlic, peppers, and Romano cheese on the mustard side. Roll up tightly and use toothpicks to secure your rolls. Transfer to the prepared baking pan.
4. Bake in the preheated oven at 370°F for about 30 minutes until golden brown on all sides (an instant-read thermometer should register 165°F).
5. Spoon the sauerkraut over the chicken and serve. Bon appétit!

Calories: 530 | Fat: 39g | Protein: 33g
Carbs: 6.7g | Net carbs: 5g | Fiber: 1.7g

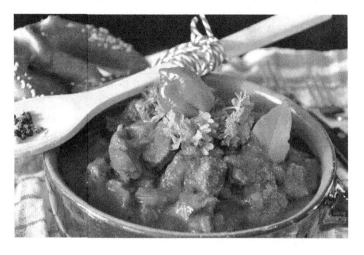

69. Turkey and Leek Goulash

Preparation time: 10 minutes | Cooking time: 40 minutes | Servings: 6

2 tablespoons olive oil
1 large-sized leek, chopped
2 cloves garlic, minced
2 pounds (907 grams) turkey thighs, skinless, boneless, and chopped
2 celery stalks, chopped

1. Heat the olive oil in a soup pot over a moderate flame. Then, sweat the leeks until just tender and fragrant.
2. Then, cook the garlic until aromatic.
3. Add in the turkey thighs and celery; add 4 cups of water and bring to a boil. Immediately reduce the
4. heat and allow it to simmer for 35 to 40 minutes. Ladle into individual bowls, serve hot. Bon appétit!

Calories: 221 | Fat: 7.3g | Protein: 35.4g
Carbs: 2.6g | Net carbs: 2.2g | Fiber: 0.4g

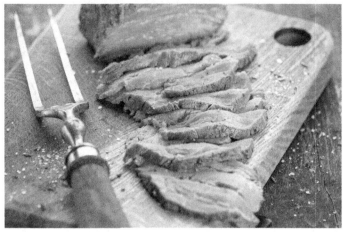

70. Beef & Broccoli Roast

Preparation time: 15 minutes | Cooking time: 4 hours 30 minutes | Servings: 2

1 pound beef chuck roast
1/2 cup beef broth
1/4 cup soy sauce
1 tbs toasted sesame oil
1 bag frozen broccoli
Pink Himalayan salt and pepper

1. With the crock insert in place, preheat your pot to low. On a cutting board, season the chuck roast with pink salt and pepper, and slice the roast thin.
2. Put the sliced beef in your pot. Combine sesame oil, soy sauce, and beef broth in a small bowl then
3. pour over the beef.
4. Cover and cook on low for 4 hours. Add the frozen broccoli and cook for 30 minutes more. If you need more liquid, add additional beef broth. Serve hot.

Calories: 803 | Carbs: 18g | Protein: 74g | Fats: 49g

Chapter 12 Snacks

71. Sweet Onion Dip

Preparation time: 15 minutes | Cooking time: 20 to 30 minutes | Servings: 2

3 cup sweet onion chopped
1/4 cup horseradish
1 teaspoon pepper sauce
2 cups mayonnaise
2 cups Swiss cheese shredded
1 tbs black pepper

1. Take a bowl, add sweet onion, horseradish, pepper sauce, mayonnaise, and Swiss cheese, mix them well and transfer them to the pie plate.
2. Preheat oven at 375°F.
3. Now, put the plate into the oven and bake for 25 to 30 minutes until the edges turn golden brown.
4. Sprinkle pepper to taste and serve with crackers.

Calories: 278 | Fat: 11.4g | Fiber: 4.1g
Carbohydrates:2.9g | Protein: 6.9g

72. Keto Trail Mix

Preparation time: 5 minutes | Cooking time: 0 minutes | Servings: 2

1/2 cup salted pumpkin seeds 1/2 cup slivered almonds
3/4 cup roasted pecan
3/4 cup unsweetened cranberries
1 cup toasted coconut flakes

1. In a skillet, place almonds and pecans. Heat for 2–3 minutes and let cool.
2. Once cooled, in a large resealable plastic bag, combine all ingredients.
3. Seal and shake vigorously to mix.
4. Evenly divide into suggested servings and store in airtight meal prep containers.

Calories: 98 | Fat: 1.2g | Fiber: 4.1g
Carbohydrates:1.1g | Protein: 3.2g

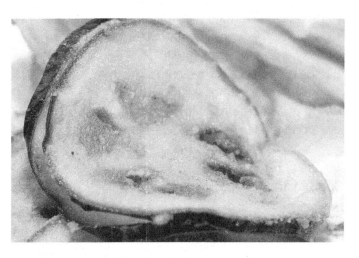

73. Eggplant Chips

Preparation time: 10 minutes | Cooking time: 20 minutes | Servings: 15

1 large eggplant, sliced
1/4 cup parmesan grated
1 teaspoon dried oregano
1/4 teaspoon dried basil
1/2 teaspoon garlic powder
1/4 cup olive oil
1/4 teaspoon pepper
1/2 teaspoon salt

1. Preheat the oven to 325°F.
2. Using a small bowl, mix oil, and dried spices.
3. Coat the eggplant with oil and spice mixture and arrange the eggplant slices on a baking tray.
4. Bake in a preheated oven for 15–20 minutes.

Calories 77 | Fat 5.8g | Carbohydrates 2g
Protein 3.5g | Sugar 0.9g | Cholesterol 8mg

74. Cold Cuts and Cheese Pinwheels

Preparation time: 20 minutes | Cooking time: 0 minutes | Servings: 5

8 ounces cream cheese, at room temperature
1/4 pound salami, sliced
2 tablespoons sliced pepperoncini

1. Sheet of plastic wrap on large on counter. Place the cream cheese in the center of the plastic
2. wrap, then add another layer of plastic wrap on top. Using a rolling pin, roll the cream cheese until it is
3. even and about 1/4 inch thick. Try to make the shape of a rectangle.
4. Pull off the top layer of plastic wrap.
5. Place the salami slices so they overlap to cover the
6. cream cheese layer completely.

7. Place a new piece of plastic wrap on top of the salami layer to flip over your cream cheese–salami rectangle. Flip the layer, the cream cheese side up.
8. Remove the wrap and add the sliced pepperoni to a layer on top.
9. Roll the layered ingredients into a tight log, pressing it together tight.
10. Then, wrap the roll with plastic wrap and refrigerate for at least 6 hours so it will be set.

Calories: 141 | Fat: 4.9g | Fiber: 2.1g
Carbohydrates: 0.3g | Protein: 8.5g

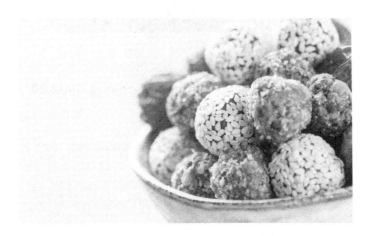

75. Strawberry Fat Bombs

Preparation time: 30 minutes | Cooking time: 0 minutes | Servings: 2

100 grams strawberries
100 grams cream cheese
50 grams butter
2 tbs erythritol powder
1/2 teaspoon vanilla extract

1. Put the cream cheese and butter (cut into small pieces) in a mixing bowl.
2. Let rest for 30 to 60 minutes at room temperature.
3. In the meantime, wash the strawberries and remove the green parts.
4. Pour into a bowl and process into a puree with a serving of oil or a mixer.
5. Add erythritol powder and vanilla extract, mix well. Mix the strawberries with the other ingredients and
6. make sure that they reached room temperature.
7. Put the cream cheese and butter into a container.
8. Mix with a hand mixer or a food processor to a homogeneous mass.
9. Pour it into small silicone muffin molds. Freeze.

Calories: 95 | Fat: 9.1g | Fiber: 4.1g
Carbohydrates: 0.9g | Protein: 2.1g

76. Zucchini Balls with Capers and Bacon

Preparation time: 3 hours | Cooking time: 20 minutes | Servings: 2

2 zucchinis, shredded
1/4 cup capers
1/2 cup grated parmesan cheese
1 garlic clove, crushed
1/2 cup cream cheese, at room temperature
2 bacon slices, chopped
1 cup Fontina cheese
1 cup crushed pork rinds
1/2 teaspoon poppy seeds
1/4 teaspoon dried dill weed
1/2 teaspoon onion powder
Salt and black pepper, to taste

1. Preheat oven to 360°F.
2. Thoroughly, mix zucchinis, capers, 1/2 of parmesan cheese, garlic, cream cheese, bacon, and Fontina cheese until well combined.
3. Shape the mixture into balls. Refrigerate 3 hours.
4. In a mixing bowl, mix the remaining parmesan
5. cheese, crushed pork rinds, dill, black pepper, onion powder, poppy seeds, and salt.
6. Roll the cheese ball in Parmesan mixture to coat. Arrange in a greased baking dish in a single layer, bake in the oven for 15–20 mins, shaking once.

Calories: 227 | Fat: 12.5g | Fiber: 9.4g
Carbohydrates: 4.3g | Protein: 14.5g

77. Parmesan and Pork Rind Green Beans

Preparation time: 5 minutes | Cooking time: 15 minutes | Servings: 2

1/2 pound green beans
2 tablespoons crushed pork rinds
2 tablespoons olive oil
1 tablespoon grated parmesan cheese
Pink Himalayan salt
Freshly ground black pepper

1. Preheat the oven to 400°F.
2. In a medium bowl, combine the green beans, pork rinds, olive oil, and parmesan cheese. Season with pink Himalayan salt and pepper, toss until the beans are thoroughly coated.
3. Spread the bean mixture on a baking sheet in single layer, roast for 15 minutes. At the halfway point, give the pan a little shake to move the beans around, or just give them a stir.

Calories: 350 | Total Fat: 30g | Carbs: 1.6g
Fiber: 6g | Protein: 8g

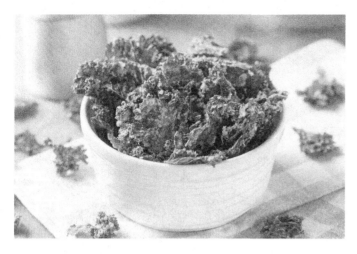

78. Kale Chips

Preparation time: 5 minutes | Cooking time: 25 minutes | Servings: 2

400 grams kale
1–2 teaspoons salt
1 tablespoon butter
50 grams bacon fat

1. Remove the stems and coarse ribs from the kale and tear the leaves into 5-centimeter pieces.
2. Wash the kale leaves thoroughly and dry them in a salad spinner.
3. Put the butter in a pan with the bacon fat and warm it up over low heat. Add salt and stir well.
4. Set aside and let cool.
5. Pack the kale in a zippered bag and pour the cooled, liquid mixture of bacon fat, & butter into it.
6. Close the zippered bag and gently shake the kale leaves with the butter mixture. The leaves should take on a glossy color due to an even film of fat.
7. Place the kale leaves on a baking sheet and sprinkle with salt, as desired.
8. Bake it for 25 minutes or until the leaves turn brown and crispy.
9. Let cool, divide into the recommended portions, and store in an airtight container.

Calories: 59 | Fat: 2.1g | Fiber: 4.5g
Carbohydrates: 0.9g | Protein: 0.4g

79. Roasted Radishes with Brown Butter Sauce

Preparation time: 10 minutes | Cooking time: 15 minutes | Servings: 2

2 cups halved radishes
1 tablespoon olive oil
Pink Himalayan salt
Freshly ground black pepper
1/2 tablespoons butter
1 tablespoon chopped fresh flat-leaf Italian parsley

1. Preheat the oven to 450°F.
2. In a medium bowl, toss the radishes in olive oil and season with pink Himalayan salt and pepper.
3. Spread the radishes on a baking sheet in a single layer. Roast for 15 minutes, stirring halfway through.
4. Meanwhile, when the radishes have been roasting for about 10 minutes, in a small, light-colored saucepan over medium heat, melt the butter completely, stirring frequently, and season with pink Himalayan salt. When the butter begins to bubble and foam, continue stirring. When the bubbling diminishes a bit, the butter should be a nice nutty brown. The browning process should take about 3 minutes total. Transfer the browned butter to a heat-safe container (I use a mug).
5. Remove the radishes from the oven, and divide them between 2 plates. Spoon the brown butter over the radishes, top with the chopped parsley, and serve.

Calories: 361 | Total Fat: 37g | Carbs: 3.8g
Fiber: 4g | Protein: 2g

80. Pesto Cauliflower Steaks

Preparation time: 5 minutes | Cooking time: 20 minutes | Servings: 2

2 tablespoons olive oil, plus more for brushing
1/2 head cauliflower
Pink Himalayan salt
Freshly ground black pepper
2 cups fresh basil leaves
1/2 cup grated parmesan cheese
1/4 cup almonds
1/2 cup shredded mozzarella cheese

1. Preheat the oven to 425°F. Brush a baking sheet with olive oil or line with a silicone baking mat. To
2. prepare the cauliflower steaks, remove and discard the leaves, and cut the cauliflower into 1-inch-thick slices. You can roast the extra floret crumbles that fall off with the steaks.

3. Place the cauliflower steaks on the prepared baking sheet, brush them with olive oil. You want the surface just lightly coated so it caramelize. Season with Himalayan salt & pepper.
4. Roast the cauliflower steaks for 20 minutes.
5. Meanwhile, put the basil, parmesan cheese, almonds, and 2 tablespoons of olive oil in a food processor (or blender), and season with pink Himalayan salt and pepper. Mix until combined.
6. Spread some pesto on top of each cauliflower steak, and top with the mozzarella cheese. Return to the oven and bake until the cheese melts, for about 2 minutes.
7. Place the cauliflower steaks on two plates, and serve hot.

Calories: 350 | Total Fat: 30g | Carbs: 1.6g
Fiber: 6g | Protein: 8g

81. Crunchy Pork Rind Zucchini Sticks

Preparation time: 5 minutes | Cooking time: 25 minutes | Servings: 2

2 medium zucchini, halved lengthwise and seeded
1/4 cup crushed pork rinds
1/4 cup grated parmesan cheese
2 garlic cloves, minced
2 tablespoons melted butter
Pink Himalayan salt
Freshly ground black pepper
Olive oil, for drizzling

1. Preheat the oven to 400°F. Line a baking sheet with aluminum foil or a silicone baking mat.
2. Place the zucchini halves cut-side up on the prepared baking sheet.
3. In a medium bowl, combine the pork rinds, parmesan cheese, garlic, and melted butter, and season with pink Himalayan salt and pepper. Mix until well combined.
4. Spoon the pork-rind mixture onto each zucchini stick, and drizzle each with a little olive oil.
5. Bake for about 20 minutes, or until the topping is golden brown.
6. Turn on the broiler to finish browning the zucchini sticks, 3 to 5 minutes, and serve.

Calories: 461 | Total Fat: 39g | Carbs: 1.5g;
Fiber: 4g | Protein: 17g

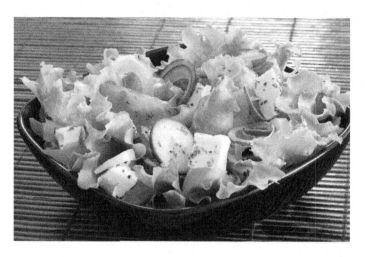

82. Tomato, Avocado, and Cucumber Salad

Preparation time: 5 minutes | Cooking time: 5 minutes | Servings: 2

1/2 cup grape tomatoes, halved
4 small Persian cucumbers or 1 English cucumber, peeled and finely chopped
1/4 cup crumbled feta cheese
1 tablespoons vinaigrette salad dressing (I use Primal Kitchen Greek Vinaigrette®)
Pink Himalayan salt
Freshly ground black pepper
1 avocado, finely chopped

1. In a large bowl, combine the tomatoes, cucumbers, avocado, and feta cheese.
2. Add the vinaigrette, and season with pink Himalayan salt and pepper. Toss to thoroughly combine.
3. Divide the salad between 2 plates and serve.

Calories: 516 | Total Fat: 45g | Carbs: 2.3g
Net Carbs: 11g | Fiber: 12g | Protein: 10g

83. Avocado Yogurt Dip

Preparation time: 5 minutes | Cooking time: 5 minutes | Servings: 4

2 avocados
1 lime juice
3 garlic cloves, minced
1/2 cup Greek yogurt
Pepper
Salt

1. Scoop out the avocado flesh using the spoon and place it in a bowl.
2. Mash avocado flesh using a fork.
3. Add the remaining ingredients and stir to mix.

Calories 139 | Fat 11g | Carbohydrates 9g
Protein 4g | Sugar 2g | Cholesterol 15 mg

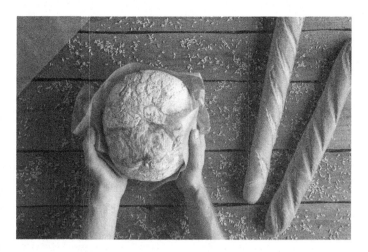

84. Keto Bread

Preparation time: 5 minutes | Cooking time: 25 minutes | Servings: 2

5 tablespoons butter, room temperature, divided	1 1/2 cups almond flour
6 eggs, lightly beaten	3 teaspoons baking powder
	Pinch pink Himalayan salt

1. Preheat the oven to 390°F. Coat a 9-by-5-inch loaf pan with 1 tablespoon of butter.
2. In a large bowl, use a hand mixer to mix the eggs, almond flour, remaining 4 tablespoons of butter, baking powder, MCT oil powder (if using), and pink Himalayan salt until thoroughly blended. Pour into the prepared pan.
3. Bake for 25 minutes, or until a toothpick inserted in the center comes out clean.

Calories: 165 | Total Fat: 178g | Carbs: 4.6g
Net Carbs: 27g | Fiber: 19g | Protein: 74g

85. Creamy Avocado Sauce

Preparation time: 5 minutes | Cooking time: 5 minutes | Servings: 8

1 avocado, halved, seeded, and peeled	2 tablespoons olive oil
1 tablespoon fresh lemon juice	3 tablespoons fresh parsley, chopped
2 garlic cloves	Pepper Salt

1. Add all ingredients into the food processor and process until smooth.
2. Serve and enjoy.

Calories 83 | Fat 8.4g | Carbohydrates 2.6g
Sugar 0.2g | Protein 0.6g | Cholesterol 0 mg

86. Loaded Cauliflower Mashed "Potatoes"

Preparation time: 10 minutes | Cooking time: 10 minutes | Servings: 2

1 head fresh cauliflower, cut into cubes	Freshly ground black pepper
2 garlic cloves, minced	1 cup shredded cheese (I use Colby Jack)
6 tablespoons butter	6 bacon slices, cooked and crumbled
1/2 tbs sour cream	
Pink Himalayan salt	

1. Boil a large pot of water over high heat. Add the cauliflower. Reduce the heat to medium-low and simmer for 8 to 10 minutes, until fork-tender. (You can also steam the cauliflower if you have a steamer basket.)
2. Drain the cauliflower in a colander, and turn it out onto a paper towel-lined plate to soak up the water. Blot to remove any remaining water from the cauliflower pieces. This step is important; you want to get out as much water as possible so the mash won't be runny.
3. Add the cauliflower to the food processor (or blender) with the garlic, butter, and sour cream, and season with pink Himalayan salt and pepper.
4. Mix for about 1 minute, stopping to scrape down the sides of the bowl every 30 seconds.
5. Divide the cauliflower mix evenly among 4 small serving dishes, and top each with the cheese and bacon crumbles. (The cheese should melt from the hot cauliflower. But if you want to reheat it, you can put the cauliflower in oven-safe serving dishes and pop them under the broiler for 1 minute to heat up the cauliflower and melt the cheese.)

Calories: 131 | Total Fat: 132g | Carbs: 3.4g
Fiber: 12g | Protein: 58g

87. Healthy Chicken Fritters

Preparation time: 10 minutes | Cooking time: 20 minutes | Servings: 4

1 1/2 pounds chicken breast, skinless, boneless, and chopped into small pieces	1 1/2 tablespoon chives, chopped
1 tablespoon olive oil	1 1/2 tablespoon fresh basil, chopped
1/2 teaspoon garlic powder	1 cup mozzarella cheese, shredded
2 tablespoons fresh parsley, chopped	1/3 cup almond flour
Salt	2 eggs, lightly beaten
	Pepper

1. Add all ingredients except oil into a large bowl and blend until well combined.
2. Heat oil in a pan over medium heat.
3. Scoop fritter mixture employing a large spoon and transfer it to the pan and cook for 6–8 minutes or until golden brown on each side.

Calories 331 | Fat 15.9g | Carbohydrates 2.9g Protein 43g | Sugar 0.6g | Cholesterol 194mg

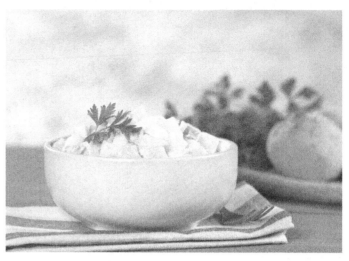

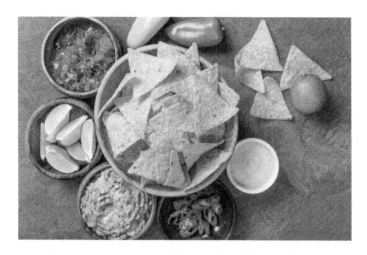

88. Cheese Chips and Guacamole

Preparation time: 10 minutes | Cooking time: 10 minutes | Servings: 2

1 cup shredded cheese
1 avocado, mashed
Juice of 1/2 lime
1 teaspoon diced jalapeño
1 tablespoon chopped fresh cilantro leaves
Pink Himalayan salt
Freshly ground black pepper

1. Preheat the oven to 350°F. Line a baking sheet with parchment paper or a silicone baking mat.
2. Add 1/4-cup of shredded cheese to the pan, leaving
3. space between them, bake until the edges are brown and the middles have melted, for 7 mins. Set the pan on a cooling rack, and let the cheese chips cool for 5 minutes. The chips will be floppy
4. when they first come out of the oven but will crisp as they cool.
5. In a medium bowl, mix together the avocado, lime juice, jalapeño, and cilantro, and season with pink Himalayan salt and pepper.
Top the cheese chips with the guacamole, serve.

Calories: 646 | Total Fat: 54g | Carbs: 1.6g
Fiber: 10g | Protein: 30g

89. Cauliflower "Potato" Salad

Preparation time: 5 minutes | Cooking time: 45 minutes | Servings: 2

1/2 head cauliflower
1 tablespoon olive oil
Pink Himalayan salt
Freshly ground black pepper
1/3 cup mayonnaise
1 tablespoon mustard
1/4 cup diced dill pickles
1 teaspoon paprika

1. Preheat the oven to 400°F. Line a baking sheet with aluminum foil or a silicone baking mat.
2. Cut the cauliflower into 1-inch pieces.
3. Put the cauliflower in a large bowl, add the olive oil, season with the pink Himalayan salt and pepper, and toss to combine.
4. Spread the cauliflower out on the prepared baking sheet and bake for 25 minutes, or just until the cauliflower begins to brown. Halfway through the cooking time, give the pan a couple of shakes or stir so all sides of the cauliflower cook.
5. In a large bowl, mix the cauliflower together with the mayonnaise, mustard, and pickles. Sprinkle the paprika on top, and chill in the refrigerator for 3 hours before serving.

Calories: 772 | Total Fat: 74g | Carbs: 2.6g
Fiber: 10g | Protein: 10g

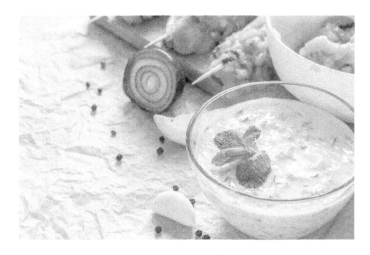

90. Perfect Cucumber Salsa

Preparation time: 5 minutes | Cooking time: 5 minutes | Servings: 10

2 1/2 cups cucumbers, peeled, seeded, chopped
2 teaspoons fresh cilantro, chopped
2 teaspoons fresh parsley, chopped
1 1/2 tablespoon fresh lemon juice
1 garlic clove, minced
1 small onion, chopped
2 large jalapeno peppers, chopped
1 1/2 cups tomatoes, chopped
1/2 teaspoon salt

1. Add all ingredients into the massive bowl and blend until well combined.

Calories 14 | Fat 0.2g | Carbohydrates 3g
Sugar 1.6g | Protein 0.6g | Cholesterol 0 mg

91. Creamy Crab Dip

Preparation time: 5 minutes | Cooking time: 5 minutes | Servings: 16

1/4 teaspoon garlic powder
2 tablespoons green onion, chopped
1 teaspoon Cajun seasoning
8 ounces crab meat
1 tablespoon lime juice
1/4 cup mayonnaise
3.5 ounces cream cheese
1/4 teaspoon pepper
1/2 teaspoon salt

1. Add all ingredients into the mixing bowl and whisk until well combined.
2. Serve and enjoy.

Calories 49 | Fat 3.6g | Carbohydrates 1.4g
Protein 2.3g | Sugar 0.3g | Cholesterol 15 mg

92. Zucchini Tots

Preparation time: 10 minutes | Cooking time: 20 minutes | Servings: 4

5 cups zucchini, grated and squeeze out all liquid
1/2 teaspoon garlic powder
1/2 teaspoon dried oregano
1/2 cup parmesan cheese, grated
1/2 cup cheddar cheese, shredded
2 eggs, lightly beaten
Pepper
Salt

1. Preheat the oven to 400°F.
2. Spray a baking tray with cooking spray and put it aside.
3. Add all ingredients into the bowl and blend until well combined.
4. Make small tots from the zucchini mixture and place them onto the prepared baking tray.
5. Bake in a preheated oven for 15–20 minutes.

Calories 353 | Fat 23.1g | Carbohydrates 9.5g
Sugar 2.8g | Protein 32.1g | Cholesterol 157 mg

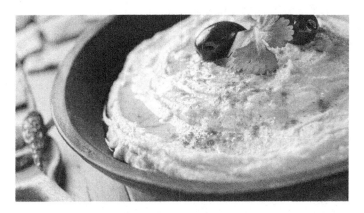

93. Keto Macadamia Hummus

Preparation time: 10 minutes | Cooking time: 5 minutes | Servings: 8

1 cup macadamia nuts, soaked in water overnight, drained and rinsed
1 1/2 tablespoon tahini
2 tablespoons water
2 tbs fresh lime juice
2 garlic cloves
1/8 teaspoon cayenne pepper
Pepper
Salt

1. Add all ingredients into the food processor and process until smooth.
2. Serve and enjoy.

Calories 138 | Fat 14.2g | Carbohydrates 3.2g
Protein 1.9g | Sugar 1.9g | Cholesterol 0mg

94. Delicious Chicken Alfredo Dip

Preparation time: 10 minutes | Cooking time: 20 minutes | Servings: 2

2 cups chicken, cooked and chopped into small pieces
1 1/2 tbs fresh parsley, chopped
1 tomato, diced
2 bacon slices, cooked and crumbled
1 1/2 cups mozzarella cheese, shredded
1 teaspoon Italian seasoning
1/2 cup parmesan cheese, grated
8 ounces cream cheese, softened
1 1/2 cups Alfredo sauce, homemade & low-carb

1. Preheat the oven to 375°F.
2. Spray a baking dish with cooking spray, put aside.
3. Add chicken, 1/2 cup mozzarella cheese, Italian seasoning, parmesan cheese, cream cheese, and Alfredo sauce to the bowl and mix.
4. Spread chicken mixture into the prepared baking dish and top with remaining mozzarella cheese.
5. Bake in a preheated oven for 20 minutes. Top with parsley, tomatoes, and bacon.

Calories 144 | Fat 0.5g | Carbohydrates 7.4g
Sugar 1.3g | Protein 29.3g | Cholesterol 216 mg

95. Easy & Perfect Meatballs

Preparation time: 10 minutes | Cooking time: 20 minutes | Servings: 8

1 egg, lightly beaten
3 garlic cloves, minced
1/2 cup mozzarella cheese, shredded
1/2 cup parmesan cheese, grated
1 pound ground beef
Pepper
Salt

1. Preheat the oven to 400°F.
2. Line a baking tray with parchment paper and put it aside.
3. Add all ingredients into the blending bowl and blend until well combined.
4. Make small balls from the meat mixture and place them on a prepared baking tray.
5. Bake in a preheated oven for 20 minutes.

Calories 157 | Fat 6.7g | Carbohydrates 0.5g
Protein 21.5g | Sugar 0.1g | Cholesterol 80 mg

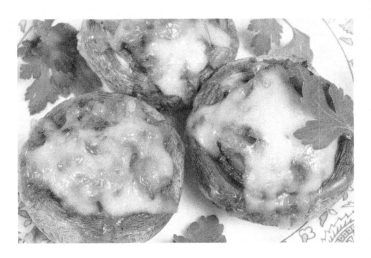

96. Cheese Stuffed Mushrooms

Preparation time: 10 minutes | Cooking time: 15 minutes | Servings: 12

12 large mushrooms, clean, remove stems and chopped stems finely
1 1/2 tbs fresh parsley, chopped
4 garlic cloves, minced
1/2 cup parmesan grated
1/4 cup Swiss cheese, grated
3.5 ounces cream cheese
1 tbs olive oil
Salt

1. Preheat the oven to 375°F.
2. Toss mushrooms with olive oil, place them onto a baking tray.
3. In a bowl, combine chopped mushrooms stems, parsley, garlic, parmesan, Swiss cheese, salt.
4. Stuff cheese mixture into the mushroom caps and arrange mushrooms on the baking tray.
Bake in a preheated oven for 10–15 minutes.

Calories 79 | Fat 6.3g | Carbohydrates 1.5g
Sugar 0.5g | Protein 4g | Cholesterol 16 mg

Chapter 13 Desserts

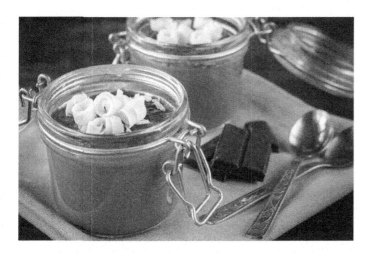

97. Chocolate Pudding Delight

Preparation time: 52 minutes | Cooking time: 0 minutes | Servings: 2

1/2 teaspoon stevia powder
2 tbs cocoa powder
2 tbs water
1 tablespoon gelatin
1 cup coconut milk
2 tbs maple syrup

1. Heat a pan with the coconut milk over medium heat; add stevia and cocoa powder and stir well.
2. In a bowl, mix gelatin with water; stir well and add to the pan.
3. Stir well, add maple syrup, whisk again, divide into ramekins and keep in the fridge for 45 minutes serve cold.

Calories: 221.2 | Total fat: 13.6g | Cholesterol: 9.8 mg
Sodium: 250.3 mg | Potassium: 86.7 mg
Total carbohydrate: 22.7g | Protein: 3.4g

98. Raspberry and Coconut

Preparation time: 15 minutes | Cooking time: 5 minutes | Servings: 12

1/4 cup swerve
1/2 cup coconut oil
1/2 cup raspberries; dried
1/2 cup coconut; shredded
1/2 cup coconut butter

1. In the food processor, blend dried berries well. Heat a pan with the butter over medium heat.
2. Add oil, coconut, and swerve; stir & cook for 5 min.
3. Pour half of this into a lined baking pan, spread.
4. Add raspberry powder and also spread.
5. Top with the rest of the butter mix, spread, and
6. keep in the fridge for a while; cut into pieces.

Carbohydrates: 45g | Sugar: 30g | Fat: 42g
Protein: 8g | Cholesterol: 0mg

99. Peanut Butter Fudge

Preparation time: 2 hours 12 minutes | Cooking time: 0 minutes | Servings: 12

1 cup peanut butter; unsweetened
1 cup coconut oil
1/4 cup almond milk
2 teaspoons vanilla stevia
A pinch of salt

For the topping
2 tablespoons swerve
1/4 cup cocoa powder
2 tablespoons melted coconut oil

1. In a heatproof bowl, mix peanut butter with coconut oil; stir and heat up in your microwave until it melts
2. Add a pinch of salt, almond milk, and stevia; stir well everything and pour into a lined loaf pan.
3. Keep in the fridge for 2 hours and then slice it.
4. In a bowl, mix melted coconut oil with cocoa powder and swerve and stir very well.
5. Drizzle the sauce over your peanut butter fudge and serve

Calories: 85 | Fat: 4.7g | Saturated fat: 2.7g
Protein: 0.5g

100. Cinnamon Streusel Egg Loaf

Preparation time: 10 minutes | Cooking time: 15 minutes | Servings: 2

2 tbs almond flour
1 tbs butter, softened
1/2 tablespoon grated butter, chilled
1 egg
1-ounce cream cheese

Others
1/2 teaspoon cinnamon, divided
1 tablespoon erythritol sweetener, divided
1/4 teaspoon vanilla extract, unsweetened

1. Turn on the oven, then set it to 350°F let it preheat. Meanwhile, crack the egg in a small bowl, add
2. cream cheese, softened butter, 1/4 teaspoon cinnamon, 1/2 tablespoon sweetener, and vanilla and whisk until well combined.
   Divide the egg batter between two silicone muffins
3. and then bake for 7 minutes.
   Meanwhile, prepare the streusel and for this, place
4. flour in a small bowl, add remaining ingredients and stir until well mixed.
5. When egg loaves have baked, sprinkle streusel on top and then continue baking for 7 minutes.
6. When done, remove loaves from the cups, let them cool for 5 minutes, serve, and enjoy!

Calories: 227 | Fat: 12.5g | Fiber: 9.4g
Carbohydrates:4.3g | Protein: 14.5g

Made in the USA
Monee, IL
11 April 2022

94566321R00066